The Hand: Fundamentals of Therapy

This book is dedicated to Kevin, Nina, Hildegard, Birger, Holger, Gunder, Ingo and Patrick

Joyce, John, Christine and Bruce

Acquisitions editor: Heidi Allen
Development editor: Myriam Brearley
Production controller: Chris Jarvis
Desk editor: Jane Campbell
Cover designer: Fred Rose

The Hand: Fundamentals of Therapy

THIRD EDITION

Judith Boscheinen-Morrin, Dip. OT, MAAOT, MAHTA
Hand Therapist, South West Hand Therapy, Sydney, Australia
(Founding Member of the Australian Hand Therapy Association)

W. Bruce Conolly, AM, FRACS, FRCS, FACS
Associate Professor, Hand Surgery, Department of Surgery, University of New South Wales, Australia.
Clinical Associate Professor, Department of Surgery, University of Sydney, Australia.
Director, Hand Unit, St Luke's Hospital, Sydney, Australia.
Staff Hand Surgeon, Hand Unit, Sydney Hospital, Sydney, Australia.

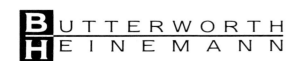

OXFORD   AUCKLAND   BOSTON   JOHANNESBURG   MELBOURNE   NEW DELHI

Butterworth-Heinemann
Linacre House, Jordan Hill, Oxford OX2 8DP
225 Wildwood Avenue, Woburn, MA 01801-2041
A division of Reed Educational and Professional Publishing Ltd

 A member of the Reed Elsevier plc group

First published 1985
Reprinted 1987, 1990
Second edition 1992
Reprinted 1995, 1997
Third edition 2001

British Library Cataloguing in Publication Data
Boscheinen-Morrin, Judith
   The hand: fundamentals of therapy – 3rd ed.
   1. Hand – Surgery – Patients – Rehabilitation
   2. Hand – Wounds and injuries – Patients – Rehabilitation
   I. Title   II. Conolly, W. Bruce
   617.5'75

Library of Congress Cataloguing in Publication Data
The hand: fundamentals of therapy/[edited by] Judith Boscheinen-Morrin,
W. Bruce Conolly. – 3rd ed.
   p.   cm.
Includes bibliographical references and index.
ISBN 0 7506 4577 6
   1. Hand – Wounds and injuries – Patients – Rehabilitation.
   2. Hand – Surgery – Patients – Rehabilitation.
   3. Hand – Diseases – Patients – Rehabilitation   4. Physical therapy.
   I. Boscheinen-Morrin, Judith.   II. Conolly, W. Bruce.
   RD559.B67
   617.5'75–dc21   00-051928

ISBN 0 7506 4577 6

Composition by Genesis Typesetting, Rochester, Kent
Printed and bound in Great Britain by The Bath Press, Avon

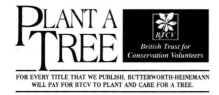

FOR EVERY TITLE THAT WE PUBLISH, BUTTERWORTH-HEINEMANN
WILL PAY FOR BTCV TO PLANT AND CARE FOR A TREE.

1

Assessment

Introduction

The hand demonstrates remarkable mobility and malleability. This allows it to conform to the multi-shaped objects that it needs to grasp (Tubiana, 1984). The hand is a unique tool of accomplishment, not only in our everyday domestic, work and leisure activities, but also in music and the arts. Just as importantly, it is an organ of expression that is used to convey emphasis and to communicate language.

The hand links us intimately to others through touch. The abundance of receptors in the skin of the palm distinguishes the hand from other areas of the body. Unlike these other areas, the hand alone is capable of simultaneously touching as it is being touched (Brun, 1963).

The hand and wrist contain 27 bones (19 miniature long bones and 8 carpal bones). There are 17 articulations involving the digits. The hand has 19 intrinsic muscles and about the same number of tendons whose origin is in the forearm.

Clinical assessment

The formulation of a treatment programme is based on a full assessment that gleans both objective and subjective data. As important as our objective findings are, Paul Brand reminds us of the need 'to balance objective assessments with trusting our impressions and to resist our tendency to reject considerations of things that we cannot quantify' (Brand, 1998). The treatment programme should therefore be tailored to the unique needs of each patient.

Most patients will require only a limited selection of all the tests that are at the therapist's disposal (Fess, 1995). Where hand pathology is complex, it is preferable to perform assessments over a number of sessions to avoid fatigue and stress. The assessment repertoire includes the following:

History

Every history begins with the patient's pertinent details, i.e. age, hand dominance, work and leisure activities and family particulars. The most important aspect of the history, however, is the reason that the patient has come for treatment. This will sometimes be obvious, e.g. after amputation of a digit or contracture associated with Dupuytren's disease. There may, however, be no obvious outward signs of injury or deformity as, for example, in patients presenting with de Quervain's disease, carpal tunnel syndrome, trigger finger or a closed wrist injury.

The history should include the following details:

1. The recency of the injury or condition.
2. The mechanism of the injury.
3. The symptoms resulting from the injury or condition and their pattern of behaviour, i.e. frequency and intensity.
4. Previous treatments and their effect.
5. Associated health problems, e.g. diabetes.
6. Prescribed medications.

Physical examination

The physical examination has both a visual and a tactile component. Much can be gleaned simply by looking at the hand. The mobility of the more proximal upper limb joints, i.e. shoulder, elbow and forearm, is assessed first. During examination, comparison is always made with the patient's other hand. It is remarkable how often features that may appear abnormal to the examiner, e.g. swan-necking, lateral deviation of a digit or joint hypermobility are normal manifestations of both hands.

Visual examination

The hand is inspected for presence of the following:

1. Wounds.
2. Scars (recent and old).
3. Swelling: where this is marked swelling there will be loss of normal skin creases (Fig. 1.1).
4. Deformity e.g. flexion deformity of the proximal interphalangeal (PIP) joint (Fig. 1.2).
5. Soft tissue contracture.
6. Muscle wasting.
7. Restricted joint motion.
8. Circulation (the hand may be pale, red or cyanosed).

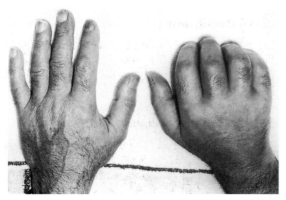

Figure 1.1. Hand oedema is common following injury. It is also associated with a number of conditions that can affect the hand. This patient developed chronic regional pain syndrome (Type 1) within weeks of surgery which involved repair of an extensor tendon. Swelling and pain were the main initial features of his condition. Note the loss of MCP joint flexion and flexed posture of the PIP joints. Note also the loss of normal skin creases over the joints.

9. Skin mottling, excessive sweating or dryness; the texture of the skin may appear smooth and shiny with loss of pulp ridging and pulp wasting; trophic lesions may be present (Fig. 1.3).
10. Nail deformity, brittleness or ridging.
11. Relevant X-rays or scans should also be viewed by the therapist (e.g. ultrasound (US), computed tomography (CT), magnetic resonance imaging (MRI)).

Tactile examination

The following are assessed by touch and will confirm much of what has been noted in the visual examination:

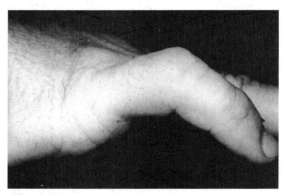

Figure 1.2. Flexion deformity at the PIP joint is the commonest deformity seen in the hand.

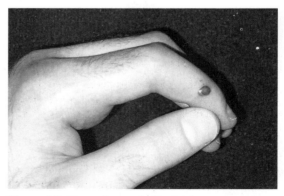

Figure 1.3. Nerve damaged skin is very prone to injury from heat, pressure, sharp objects or friction. Note the smooth, shiny skin of the thumb and index finger following injury to the median nerve.

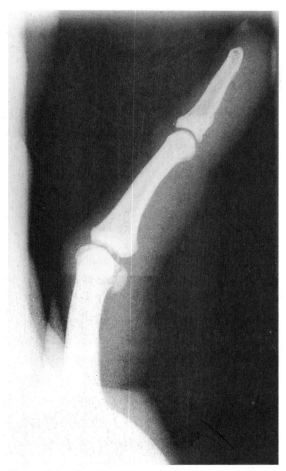

Figure 1.4. All relevant X-ray findings and results from diagnostic tests, e.g. nerve conduction studies, ultrasound, bone scans, magnetic resonance imaging, etc., should be recorded in the patient's history.

1. Scar condition

Palpation of the scar will determine areas of hypersensitivity and whether the scar is supple and mobile or rigid and adherent.

2. Temperature of the skin

Increased temperature may indicate inflammation/ infection or early-stage chronic regional pain syndrome (CRPS); decreased temperature may be a sign of poor circulation (e.g. Raynaud's disease), nerve injury or later-stage CRPS.

3. Swelling

The skin is indented to determine whether oedema is soft and yielding (usually acute) or 'woody' and dense (subacute or chronic).

4. Thickenings or nodules

The palm is palpated for thickenings or nodules that are not apparent on visual inspection, e.g. thickening of the A1 pulley (trigger finger) or tight fascial bands or nodules that may indicate early Dupuytren's disease.

5. Soft tissue tightness

The forearm and hand are palpated for soft tissue tightness that may be limiting movement at the wrist and/or finger joints, e.g. following nerve and flexor tendon repair at the wrist, protracted flexion splinting can result in muscle-tendon shortening. Adherence of tendons can also affect the hand's normal tenodesis effect whereby flexion of the wrist will facilitate finger extension and conversely, extension of the wrist will facilitate finger flexion.

6. Moistness or dryness of the skin

Excessive sweating (hyperhidrosis) is normal in some patients; however, it can be a sign of CRPS; excessive dryness is a feature of nerve damage.

7. Joint stiffness

Joints are passively moved to determine whether they have a 'springy' or 'hard' end-feel; generally, the latter does not augur well for conservative treatment outcome.

8 Palpation of the hand

This may identify painful areas, e.g. where there is a neuroma, an arthritic joint or tendonitis.

Pain

Pain is difficult to assess clinically because its experience is unique to each individual. The patient is asked to describe the nature of the pain, i.e. stabbing, burning, shooting or aching. The patient should indicate whether the pain is localized or radiating and whether it is deep or superficial. The intensity, duration and sources of provocation are also recorded (Echternach, 1993).

Acute postinjury or postoperative pain is to be anticipated and generally passes uneventfully. Pain that persists can be 'graded' on a linear pain scale of 0–10, with '0' representing no pain and '10' representing the severest level of pain. This visual analogue scale (VAS) can be used before and after treatment sessions as a guide to determine the efficacy of treatment.

Range of motion

Range of motion can be determined in a number of ways (Cambridge-Keeling, 1995). In everyday clinical practice, both active (AROM) and passive range of motion (PROM) should be recorded, bearing in mind that the active motion of the joint will be limited by the joint's passive capacity. This information is important in determining whether treatment measures are achieving the desired result, e.g. in the case of corrective splinting. Range of motion is also recorded to compare pre- and postoperative results.

Rigorous recording is less relevant in conditions where improvement in ROM is anticipated, e.g. in the acutely swollen digit or hand where an increase in joint mobility occurs inevitably as oedema is resolved.

1. Active range of motion (AROM)

This refers to the arc of motion that is achieved when the muscles that control a joint are used to move it. Causes of limited active range of motion can include: loss of tendon continuity, tendon adhesion (e.g. following repair or significant injury), tendon inflammation (e.g. rheumatoid disease or overuse), tendon constriction (e.g. trigger finger or de Quervain's disease), tendon subluxation or dislocation.

2. Passive range of motion (PROM)

This refers to the arc of motion that is achieved when an external force, such as the examiner's hand, is used to move the joint. Factors that can influence a joint's passive range include disruption of the articular surfaces (intra-articular fracture) and/or capsular fibrosis, e.g. after prolonged immobilization.

3. Total active range of motion (TAROM)

This refers to the total flexion range of a digit when its three joints are flexed simultaneously and any extension deficit over the three digital joints is subtracted.

4. Total passive range of motion (TPROM)

As for TAROM except that an external force is used to move the digit.

5. Composite finger flexion to the palm

This measures the distance of the finger pulp from the palm when all three finger joints are flexed simultaneously. Where flexion range is near-normal, the finger pulp will lie over the distal palmar crease. Where flexion range is more restricted, the finger pulp will lie over the mid- or proximal-palm area (Fig. 1.5).

6. Torque range of motion (TROM)

Torque range of motion involves moving a joint passively through its range of motion using a constant force. The objective of torque angle range of motion is to provide a more objective PROM assessment (Brand, 1993). To measure the force applied during passive motion, Brand advocates the use of a Haldex gauge, a spring scale or a push-pull device calibrated in grams up to one kilogram. Breger-Lee and others (1990) also use the Haldex gauge and in their research have noted that higher force levels, i.e. around 800 g, provide more consistent correlations during interphalangeal joint measurements.

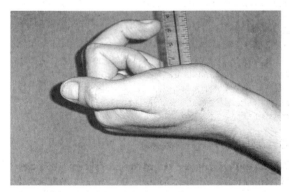

Figure 1.5. Composite finger flexion can be assessed with a ruler that measures the distance from the pulp of the finger to the palm.

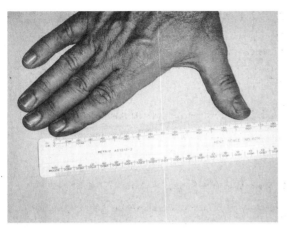

Figure 1.6. Thumb web span or interdigital span can be measured with a ruler.

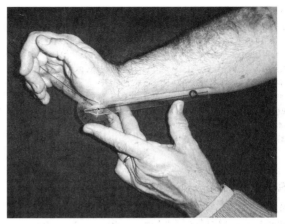

Figure 1.7. The size of the goniometer should be appropriate to the joint being measured. For wrist and forearm assessment, the goniometer will require an arm of at least 15 cm in length.

7. Thumb or finger web spans

These can be measured with a ruler by determining the distance between the tips of the various digits (Fig. 1.6).

Assessment of motion with a goniometer

Joint range of motion can be reliably assessed with a goniometer (Hellebrandt et al., 1949). The size of the goniometer should be appropriate to the joint being measured. The arm of the goniometer used to measure the wrist and forearm is about 15 cm in length compared to the 4–6 cm arm needed to assess digital range of motion (Fig. 1.7).

Positioning of the hand during measuring

The position of the forearm and hand should be consistent during each recording. When measuring finger joint ROM, the wrist should be held in neutral and the forearm in pronation. This position eliminates the possibility of restricted tendon glide due to the tenodesis effect, i.e. restriction of finger flexion when the wrist is maximally flexed and restriction of finger extension when the wrist is maximally extended.

Goniometer placement

To minimize intertester error, a specific protocol should be adopted (Hamilton and Lachenbruch, 1969). The goniometer can be placed laterally or dorsally. The author believes that there is less margin for error in dorsal placement and therefore

prefers this method. It is important that the fulcrum is centred over the joint and that the arms of the goniometer lie over the long axes of the adjacent bones. To ensure optimum accuracy, the contact of the goniometer arms with the skin should be as intimate as possible (Perry and Bevin, 1974) (Fig. 1.8).

When measuring flexion range of the distal interphalangeal joint (DIP) joint during global flexion, proper placement of the goniometer is not always possible. The patient is therefore asked to slightly extend the metacarpophalangeal (MCP) joints to accommodate goniometer placement. Full extension at these joints, i.e. a hook grip, will best facilitate measurement of the DIP joints.

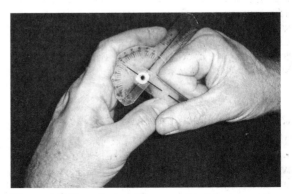

Figure 1.8. To optimize accuracy when assessing range of motion, the contact of the goniometer arms with the skin should be as intimate as possible.

Method of recording

Range of motion is usually expressed as extension/flexion, with 0 degrees regarded as neutral. For example, 20/105 degrees of active movement at the PIP joint of the right index finger would denote a 20 degree flexion deformity and 105 degrees of flexion. In other words, a total active range of 85 degrees. If the minus sign appears before extension range, i.e. −20/105, this would denote a 20 degree range of hyperextension at the PIP joint.

Oedema assessment

Oedema can be assessed simply with a tape measure that is applied at specific anatomical landmarks, e.g. at the PIP joint of the single digit or around the MCP joints when assessing hand oedema (Fig. 1.9).

In everyday clinical practice, the assessment of hand or finger swelling has little relevance. In most cases, oedema subsides uneventfully in response to simple measures such as elevation, light compression bandaging and the commencement of early active movement where this is not contraindicated.

If oedema is noted to fluctuate for no apparent reason, there may be an indication for formally recording these changes. This fluctuation may indicate an impending pain syndrome or rarely, the patient may be deliberately perpetuating a swollen hand for secondary gain.

A more formal method of measuring changes to oedema is by means of water displacement when the hand is immersed in a large Perspex container, such as the 'Volumeter' designed by Dr Paul Brand and Helen Wood, OTR. in Louisiana (Waylett-Rendall and Seibly, 1991). The tank is filled to a known level and the hand and wrist are held vertically and placed into the tank to a predetermined level marked circumferentially on the forearm. When the water settles after rising, the difference in volume is recorded.

Sensibility testing

Cutaneous sensibility refers to the conscious appreciation and interpretation of a tactile stimulus (Fig. 1.10). Objective assessment of sensibility is difficult. This is due in part to the subjective responses of the patient and to the fact that there is considerable variation in the application of force and velocity during hand-held examination techniques (Bell-Krotoski and Buford, 1988). Even the results of nerve conduction velocity tests can be influenced by factors such as the size and placement of electrodes, temperature of the extremity and even the time of the day that testing occurs.

The reasons for assessing sensibility include:

1. To determine the extent of sensory loss following a nerve lesion.
2. To assist in the diagnosis of neuropathies, e.g. carpal tunnel syndrome.
3. To determine the most suitable time to initiate sensory re-education (i.e. upon return of moving touch).
4. To monitor recovery of sensibility after nerve repair.
5. To help determine the degree of functional impairment for medicolegal purposes.

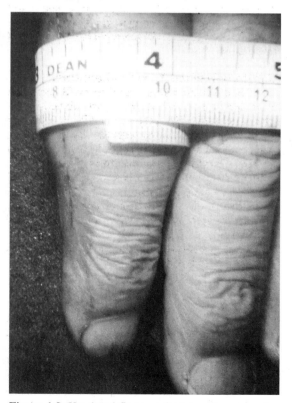

Figure 1.9. Hand and finger oedema can be assessed with a tape measure that is applied at specific anatomical landmarks, e.g. at the PIP joint.

Types of tests

Because no single test can adequately assess sensibility, a battery of tests should be used

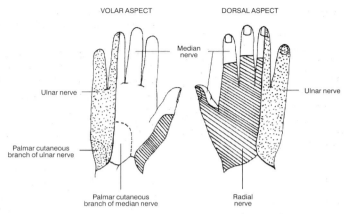

VOLAR ASPECT   DORSAL ASPECT

Median
nerve

Ulnar nerve   Ulnar nerve

Palmar cutaneous
branch of ulnar nerve

Palmar cutaneous   Radial
branch of median nerve   nerve

Figure 1.10. Sensory distribution in the hand showing the areas of median, ulnar and radial nerve innervation.

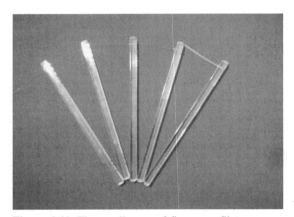

Figure 1.11. The smaller set of five monofilaments represents the highest calculated force of each functional sensory level and can be used without sacrificing test sensitivity.

(Callahan, 1995). This will help determine not only sensory acuity, but also how acuity relates to functional ability (Bell-Krotoski, 1995; Clark, 1999). Sensibility tests can be divided into various categories, e.g. threshold tests, innervation density tests, tactile gnosis tests or objective tests.

1. Threshold tests

The two threshold tests are vibration and touch-pressure (Semmes-Weinstein monofilaments). The monofilament test is helpful in monitoring return of sensibility following nerve repair. Both tests are used to detect the gradual change in nerve function that occurs in compression syndromes (Dellon, 1980) and that does not involve cortical integration (Szabo, 1999). When assessing compression syndromes, other sensibility tests, such as static and moving two-point discrimination (which are innervation density tests), will not register changes until much later.

Semmes-Weinstein monofilaments

The 'light touch-deep pressure' monofilament test is regarded as one of the most objective for cutaneous sensibility assessment (Table 1). Light touch sensibility is a prerequisite for performing fine discriminatory tasks while deep pressure is a form of protective sensation. Based on von Frey's pressure sensibility test for warmth, cold, pain and touch, Semmes, Weinstein and others (1960) developed a testing instrument to assess somatosensory changes in adults following brain damage. This testing system was then adopted by von Prince for assessment of the nerve-injured hand (von Prince and Butler, 1967).

The full testing kit includes 20 colour-coded nylon filaments, each mounted in a Lucite rod. The monofilaments are calibrated to exert specific pressures. The lightest monofilament exerts a 4.5 mg force while the heaviest filament exerts a 447 g force. A smaller set of five monofilaments represents the highest calculated force of each functional sensory level (i.e. normal, diminished light touch, diminished protective sensation and loss of protective sensation) and can be used without sacrificing test sensitivity (Bell-Krotoski, 1993) (Fig. 1.11).

Table 1.1. Semmes-Weinstein monofilament scale of interpretation

Filament	Interpretation	Force (g)
1.65–**2.83*** (Green)	Normal light touch	0.0045–0.068
3.22–**3.61** (Blue)	Diminished light touch	0.166–0.408
3.84–**4.31** (Purple)	Diminished protective sensation	0.696–2.052
4.56–**6.65** (Red)	Loss of protective sensation	3.63–447
Greater than 6.65 (Red-lined)	Untestable (no response)	Greater than 447

*Miniset monofilaments are in bold.

Technique

This test requires the patient's full concentration and should therefore be carried out in a quiet environment, free of distractions. Because nerve conduction velocity is slowed with low temperatures (de Jesus et al., 1973), the testing room should be warm, as should the patient's hand during testing. The hand is stabilized (exercise putty is ideal for this purpose) and vision is occluded (Fig. 1.12).

The area of sensory dysfunction is mapped out and the test is begun with filament 2.83. The examiner can commence the test with a higher numbered filament where sensibility is very poor. Each filament is applied to the skin perpendicularly for 1–1.5 s until it bends. The filament is held for 1–1.5 s and then lifted in the same timeframe. Each filament is applied to the same spot on three occasions. An affirmative response is recorded if one of the three applications elicits a response. The response is then recorded on the grid pattern with the appropriate colour and dated for later comparison (Fig. 1.13).

When monitoring progressive nerve compression, all relevant areas of nerve distribution should be assessed. For other conditions, e.g. following nerve repair, testing can be confined to the volar digital pulps where receptor density is most concentrated (Moran, 1981).

2. Innervation density tests

Static two-point discrimination, moving two-point discrimination and localization are innervation density tests (also referred to as functional tests) that require complex cortical integration. Two-point discrimination is considered to relate to the hand's ability to perform fine tasks such as winding a watch or threading a needle (Moberg, 1958). Instruments used for this test include the Boley Gauge, the 'Disk-Criminator' or a paper clip. This test is only relevant in the tips of the fingers where discrimination is required (Fig. 1.14).

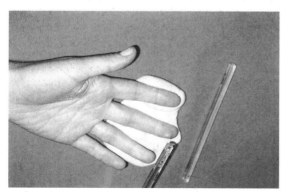

Figure 1.12. The hand can be effectively stabilized with putty during monofilament testing.

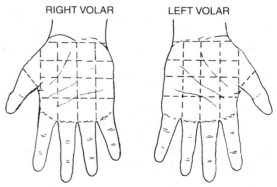

RIGHT VOLAR   LEFT VOLAR

Figure 1.13. Grid pattern for recording results of monofilament testing of light touch-deep pressure sensibility.

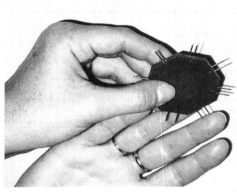

Figure 1.14. The 'Disk-Criminator' is used to test two-point discrimination in the tips of the fingers.

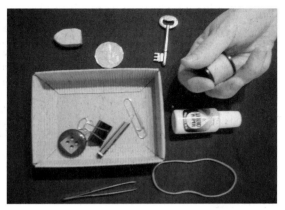

Figure 1.15. The 'pick-up test' is a test of tactile gnosis that requires some motor dexterity. The patient picks up a number of objects as quickly as possible and places them in a box. The procedure is timed and comparison is made with the opposite hand.

Table 1.2. Two-point discrimination in the hand*

Pulp of the thumb	2.5–5 mm
Pulp of the index finger	3–5 mm
Pulps of the other digits	4–6 mm
Base of the palmar aspect of the digits	5–6 mm
Thenar and hypothenar eminences	5–9 mm
Midpalmar region	11 mm
Dorsal aspect of the digits	6–9 mm
Dorsal aspect of the hand	7–12 mm

*After Tubiana, 1984.

Table 1.3. Two-point discrimination norms*

Normal	Less than 6 mm
Fair	6–10 mm
Poor	11–15 mm
Protective	One point perceived
Anaesthetic	No points perceived

*American Society for Surgery of the Hand Guidelines.

(a) Static two-point discrimination

With vision occluded, the test is commenced with a point-to-point distance of 5 mm. The points are applied longitudinally with minimal pressure that should not cause blanching. To record an accurate response, 7 out of 10 responses must be correct. The distance between the points is increased by 1, 2 or 5 mm if the response is incorrect (Callahan, 1995).

(b) Moving two-point discrimination

When assessing moving two-point discrimination, testing is carried out in a proximal to distal direction with the instrument initially set at a distance of 8 mm (Dellon, 1978). Following nerve repair, return of moving two-point discrimination precedes static two-point discrimination by several months.

(c) Point localization

Point localization is assessed using the lowest numbered filament that the patient is able to perceive during light touch testing. With vision occluded, the filament is applied to the hand. The patient is then asked, with eyes open, to identify the point of contact with the other hand. The correct response is then recorded with a dot on a grid pattern such as that used for recording light touch. Where the response is incorrect, the grid is marked with an arrow from the point of stimulation to the area where the touch has been referred (head of arrow). As sensibility improves, follow-up testing should show fewer and shorter arrows (Callahan, 1983).

3. Tactile gnosis tests

These tests require active patient participation and involve everyday objects such as a key, coin, safety pin, paper clip, screw, marble, nuts and bolts. The Moberg pickup test (Moberg, 1958) and Dellon's modification of this test (1981) require the patient to pick up objects as quickly as possible and place them into a box while sighting the objects (Fig. 1.15). This procedure is timed and comparison is made with the uninvolved hand. If the patient lacks the ability to manipulate the objects because of poor motor function, the test is discontinued.

Where motor dexterity is adequate to perform the test, it is repeated, this time with vision occluded. Note is taken of the manner in which the patient handles the objects, i.e. areas of the hand that are not used due to poor sensibility. Dellon standardized the original test items by choosing objects of a similar material (i.e. all metallic) to avoid providing clues that can be gained through variation in texture and temperature.

4. Objective tests

These tests include the Ninhydrin sweat test and wrinkle test and require no patient participation as they rely on a sympathetic response. The sweat test identifies areas of disturbed sweat secretion and can be carried out with commercially available Ninhydrin developer and fixer. The wrinkle test involves placing the hand in warm water (40°C) for a period of 30 min (O'Rain, 1973).

These tests are considered useful in the assessment of children, patients who are unable to comply with formal testing or those suspected of malingering. While these tests can be indicative of sensory function, their results do not correlate directly with sensibility during nerve regeneration, while in the case of nerve compression syndromes, there is no correlation (Phelps and Walker, 1977).

Tinel's sign

Nerve regeneration can be monitored by Tinel's sign which was described in 1915 by both Tinel and Hoffman. The paraesthesia (i.e. pins and needles) experienced by the patient when the nerve is percussed is caused by regeneration of the sensory axons which are very sensitive to pressure.

According to Tinel, the sign appears about 4 to 6 weeks after injury, although this timeframe can vary significantly according to the severity of the lesion. While the test has limited functional value (it can be elicited even where there are only few regenerating fibres), it is useful in confirming axonal growth.

Technique

Using the tip of the finger, the examiner gently percusses along the course of the nerve in a distal to proximal direction. Percussion is continued until paraesthesia is elicited. This sensation, whilst unpleasant, is not painful and should be felt peripherally in the cutaneous distribution of the nerve rather than at the point of direct pressure.

The test is repeated every few weeks. A good prognosis is suggested where distal progression of the sign is noted. Tinel's sign should be interpreted in the light of other clinical findings.

Grip strength measurement

1. Power grip

Power grip strength can be reliably assessed with the Jamar dynamometer (Bechtol, 1954) on the condition that calibration of the instrument is maintained. The dynamometer has five handle positions, each of which influence the strength of

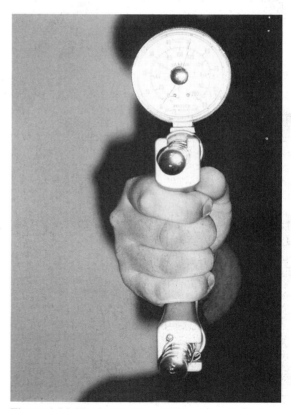

Figure 1.16. The Jamar dynamometer is a reliable tool for assessing grip strength. The test is performed with the shoulder adducted, the elbow flexed to 90 degrees, the forearm in neutral rotation and the wrist in 0–30 degrees of extension and slight ulnar deviation.

grip (Fig. 1.16). Readings diminish in the following 'handle position' order: third (strongest), second, fourth, fifth and first (Fess, 1982).

The testing position is as follows: shoulder adducted, elbow flexed to 90 degrees, forearm in neutral rotation, wrist between 0 to 30 degrees of extension and in slight ulnar deviation. The 'second handle' position was recommended as the test position in 1978 by the 'Clinical Assessment Committee of the American Society for Surgery of the Hand'. The test is performed three times with a short rest period allowed between readings so that the result is not affected by fatigue. The average of the readings is then recorded.

A patient is suspected of fudging the results if:

1. The readings are quite erratic, i.e. the discrepancy is greater than 20 per cent (it may be much higher).
2. The normal bell curve of grip strength, that is noted when testing in each of the five positions, is absent; the result will be a flat curve with each of the readings being very similar (Aulicino, 1995).

2. Pinch grip strength

Pinch grip strength is assessed with a pinch gauge which assesses (1) tip-to-tip pinch between the thumb and index finger (weakest pinch), (2) lateral pinch where the thumb is clasped against the radial side of the index finger (strongest pinch grip) and (3) three-jaw chuck where the pulp of the thumb is pinched against the pulps of the

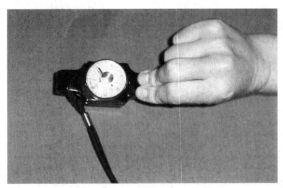

Figure 1.17. A pinch gauge is used to assess the three pinch grip positions: (1) tip-to-tip pinch between the thumb and index finger; (2) lateral (or key) pinch between the thumb and radial aspect of the index finger; (3) three-jaw chuck pinch between the thumb and index and middle fingers (as above).

index and middle fingers. As for power grip, the test is repeated three times and the average reading is recorded (Fig. 1.17).

Manual muscle testing

Manual muscle testing (Kendall et al., 1971) is indicated in the following circumstances:

1. To determine precisely which muscles have been affected following a nerve lesion.
2. As a preoperative evaluation in determining which muscles can be utilized for tendon transfer.
3. In helping to monitor motor progress during nerve regeneration.

Grading of strength is as follows:

0. No evidence of contraction.
1. Evidence of slight muscle contraction; no joint movement.
2. Muscle contraction producing movement with gravity eliminated.
3. Muscle contraction producing movement against gravity.
4. Muscle contraction producing movement against gravity with some resistance.
5. Muscle contraction producing movement against full resistance.

Functional assessment

The patient is assessed for any problems relating to routine activities of daily living (ADL). Where indicated, aids can be provided on a temporary basis to encourage early use of the hand. The commonest aid involves the enlargement of small handles, e.g. cutlery, toothbrush or razor, to enable grasp.

Complex injuries or conditions such as rheumatoid arthritis will require full functional assessments involving all aspects of the patient's life, i.e. home, work and leisure. These assessments may need to be carried out at regular intervals as the patient's functional status alters.

Psychological assessment

The hand and psyche are inextricably linked (Grant, 1980). The psychological responses following hand trauma vary considerably and can be complex. To some patients, altered body image results in serious loss of self-esteem and emotional disturbance. Others are more affected by potential loss of function and what this will mean in relation to work and recreational activities. An individual's reaction to injury is not always in proportion to the extent of physical damage. Cultural factors may play an important role as does a patient's premorbid personality or pre-existing psychological problems.

Where injury to the hand has been serious, the repercussions for the patient can be enormous. Apart from the possible financial implications of being unable to work, the dynamics of the patient's family and social life are also radically altered. The mental/emotional state of the patient should be monitored closely for persisting signs of anxiety and/or depression. While these reactions are normal in the short term, their persistence should be taken seriously and appropriate psychiatric intervention should be arranged.

References

Aulicino, P. L. (1995). Clinical examination of the hand. In *Rehabilitation of the Hand: Surgery and Therapy* (J. M. Hunter, E. J. Mackin and A. D. Callahan, eds) pp. 53–75, Mosby.

Bechtol, C. D. (1954). Grip test: use of a dynamometer with adjustable handle spacing. *J. Bone Joint Surg.,* **36A**, 820.

Bell-Krotoski, J. (1993). 'Pocket filaments' and specifications for the Semmes-Weinstein monofilaments. *J. Hand Ther.,* **3(1)**, 26–9.

Bell-Krotoski, J. (1995). Sensibility testing: current concepts. In *Rehabilitation of the Hand: Surgery and Therapy* (J. M. Hunter, E. J. Mackin and A. D. Callahan, eds) pp. 109–28, Mosby.

Bell-Krotoski, J. and Buford, W. Jr. (1988). The force/time relationship of clinically used sensory testing instruments. *J. Hand Ther.,* **1(2)**, 76.

Brand, P. W. (1993). Methods of clinical measurement of the hand. In *Clinical Mechanics of the Hand*, 2nd edn (P. W. Brand and A. Hollister, eds) pp. 223–53, Mosby Year Book.

Brand, P. W. (1998). The mind and spirit in hand therapy. *J. Hand Ther.,* **1(4)**, 145–7.

Breger-Lee, D., Bell-Krotoski, J. and Brandsma, J. (1990). Torque range of motion in the hand clinic. *J. Hand Ther.,* **3**, 7–13.

Brun, J. (1963). *La Main et l'Esprit*. Presses Universitaires de France.

Callahan, A. D. (1984) Sensibility testing: clinical methods. In *Rehabilitation of the Hand: Surgery and Therapy*, 2nd edn (J. M. Hunter, L. H. Schneider, E. J. Mackin and A. D. Callahan, eds) pp. 407–31, Mosby.

Callahan, A. D. (1995). Sensibility assessment: prerequisites and techniques for nerve lesions in continuity and nerve lacerations. In *Rehabilitation of the Hand: Surgery and Therapy* (J. M. Hunter, E. J. Mackin and A. D. Callahan, eds) pp. 129–52, Mosby.

Cambridge-Keeling, C. A. (1995). Range-of-motion measurement of the hand. In *Rehabilitation of the Hand: Surgery and Therapy* (J. M. Hunter, E. J. Mackin and A. D. Callahan, eds) pp. 93–107, Mosby.

Clark, T. (1999). Digital nerve repair: the relationship between sensibility and dexterity. Thesis (MSc. – Coursework), Curtin University of Technology.

de Jesus, P., Hausmanow-Petruse-Wics, I. and Barchi, R. (1973). The effect of cold on nerve conduction of human slow and fast nerve fibers. *Neurology,* **23**, 1182.

Dellon, A. L. (1978). The moving two-point discrimination test: clinical evaluation of the quickly-adapting fiber/receptor system *J. Hand Surg.,* **3**, 474.

Dellon, A. L. (1980). Clinical use of vibratory stimuli to evaluate peripheral nerve injury and compression neuropathy. *Plast. Reconstr. Surg.,* **65**, 466.

Dellon, A. L. (1981). *Evaluation of Sensibility and Re-education of Sensation in the Hand*. Williams & Wilkins.

Echternach, J. L. (1993). Clinical evaluation of pain. *Phys. Ther. Prac.,* **2(3)**, 14–26.

Fess, E. E. (1982). The effects of Jamar dynamometer handle position and test protocol on normal grip strength. Procedures of the American Society of Hand Therapists. *J. Hand Surg.,* **7**, 308.

Fess, E. E. (1995). Documentation: Essential elements of an upper extremity assessment battery. In *Rehabilitation of the Hand: Surgery and Therapy* (J. M. Hunter, E. J. Mackin and A. D. Callahan, eds) pp. 185–214, Mosby.

Grant, G. H. (1980). The hand and the psyche. *J. Hand Surg.,* **5**, 417–9.

Hamilton, G. F. and Lachenbruch, P. A. (1969). The reliability of goniometry in assessing finger joint angle. *Phys. Ther.,* **49**, 465.

Hellebrandt, F. A., Duvall, E. N. and Moore, M. L. (1949). The measurement of joint motion. Part III. Reliability of goniometry. *Phys. Ther. Rev.,* **29**, 302.

Kendall, H, Kendall, F. and Wadsworth, G. (1971). *Muscle Testing and Function*. Williams & Wilkins.

Moberg, E. (1958). Objective methods for determining the functional value of sensitivity in the hand. *J. Bone Joint Surg.,* **40B**, 454–76.

Moran, C. (1981). Comparison of sensory testing methods using carpal tunnel syndrome patients. Unpublished Masters Thesis. Medical College of Virginia, Virginia Commonwealth University.

O'Rain, S. (1973). New and simple test for nerve function in the hand. *Br. Med. J.,* **3**, 615.

Perry, J. F. and Bevin, A. G. (1974). Evaluation procedures for patients with hand injuries. *Phys. Ther.,* **54**, 593.

Phelps, P. and Walker, E. (1977). Comparison of the finger wrinkling test results to establish sensory tests in peripheral nerve injury. *Am. J. Occ. Ther.,* **31**, 565.

Semmes, J., Weinstein, S., Ghent, L. and Teaber, H. L. (1960). *Somatosensory Changes after Penetrating Brain Wounds in Man.* Harvard University Press.

Szabo, R. M. (1999). Entrapment and compression neuropathies. In *Green's Operative Hand Surgery* (D. P. Green, R. N. Hotchkiss and W. C. Pederson, eds) pp. 1404–47, Churchill Livingstone.

Tinel, J. (1915). Le signe du 'fourmillement' dans les lesions des nerfs peripheriques. *Press. Med.,* **47**, 388–9.

Tubiana, R. (1984). Architecture and functions of the hand. In *Examination of the Hand and Upper Limb* (R. Tubiana, ed.) pp. 1–97, W. B. Saunders.

von Prince, K. and Butler, B. (1967). Measuring sensory function of the hand in peripheral nerve injuries. *Am. J. Occ. Ther.,* **21**, 385.

Waylett-Rendall, J. and Seibly, D. (1991). A study of the accuracy of a commercially available volumeter. *J. Hand Ther.,* **4(1)**, 10–3.

2

Treatment principles and tools

Introduction

Care of the hand following injury or surgery aims to restore function without compromising the healing process. To formulate an aftercare programme, the therapist needs to appreciate the various phases of wound healing and the implications for treatment that are inherent in each of these phases.

Phases of wound healing

No matter what the wound type, the healing process is achieved by a series of complex events that are interlinked and interdependent. Wound healing can be influenced by many factors: infection, disease (e.g. diabetes), the effect of drugs (e.g. steroids), pain, cold exposure or emotional stress (Hunt and Hussain, 1992). Where healing is uncomplicated, the timetable of these events is fairly predictable. The three phases of healing are:

1. The inflammatory or exudative phase (the first 3 to 4 days)

The inflammatory phase is characterized by oedema, redness, heat and pain. The oedema resulting from injury is different to that associated with medical conditions such as chronic heart failure, kidney disease or postmastectomy lymphoedema (Hardy, 1986). The oedema associated with these conditions is referred to as 'transudate' and is caused by increased hydrostatic pressure. This oedema is low in protein (Witte and Witte, 1971) and causes minimal fibroplasia. The potential for adhesion formation is therefore negligible.

Injury to the hand, however, causes disruption of capillary integrity. The exudate that leaks from damaged vessels is a protein fluid that is rich in fibroblasts. Propensity for adhesion is therefore high. Where the inflammatory phase of healing is prolonged through careless wound handling or too early or vigorous movement, increased fibroplasia and scarring can ensue.

At the time of injury, blood flow is arrested by a short period of vasoconstriction. This is followed by vasodilation when histamine is released into the injured area and there is an increase in blood flow and the leaking of plasma into the wound region. This inflammatory exudate causes pain, partly through tissue distension and partly from irritation of the nerve endings by substances contained within the exudate, e.g. prostaglandins (Peacock, 1984).

Blood flow then ceases as a result of platelet aggregation. This clotting process precipitates fibrin formation and the creation of a network of fibres that joins the sides of the wound together. Devitalized tissue and debris is then cleared from the wound by leuocytes and macrophages in a process known as phagocytosis (Smith, 1995). This is followed by the growth of new capillary buds that bridge the wound.

The surface of the wound is usually covered by the third day as epithelial cells migrate into the wound from the basal layers of the epidermis. This migration follows converging paths from every part of the wound edge. When the migrating cells meet each other, they stop moving due to a recognition process called 'contact inhibition'. They then continue to divide, thereby restoring the thickness of the epidermis. The mitotic rate of epithelial cells at the wound surface is about 40 times higher than that of uninjured tissue (Hugo, 1977). Wound cover prevents fluid loss and provides a barrier against infection (Peacock, 1984).

Aims of treatment

(a) To protect the vulnerability of the wound

Wounds should be covered with dressings that prevent fluids escaping from the wound bed. Maintenance of wound humidity enhances cellular activity (Alvarez, 1989) and advances the process of angiogenesis. The newer 'microenvironmental' dressings, e.g. Tegaderm, Lyofoam, Intrasite and Duoderm, are used for specific types of wound and maintain an environment that promotes healing. The wound is further protected with supportive bandaging or splinting. Dressings that tend to dehydrate, e.g. the paraffin gauzes, are difficult and painful to remove (particularly in the case of fingertip injuries) and can disrupt or retard the healing process.

(b) To reduce pain

Dressings that maintain wound humidity decrease pain and reduce mechanical trauma when the dressing is removed. Supportive splinting and elevation will help reduce pain by relieving tissue distension. Short-term use of analgesics may be indicated.

(c) To promote resolution of oedema

To minimize the potential for fibrosis and scarring, oedema reduction is a priority after injury or surgery. This is achieved with gentle compressive dressings and elevation above heart level. Where appropriate, gentle active finger movement is commenced.

2. Fibroplastic or regenerative phase

This phase of healing begins after about the 5th day and can last from 2 to 6 weeks depending on the extent of the wound. The key cell during this phase is the fibroblast. This is a connective tissue cell that synthesizes and secretes collagen and other intercellular substances required to produce new tissue. The formation of granulation tissue is dependent on a network of blood vessels being formed in the injured tissue bed (i.e. angiogenesis). A capillary network has usually formed by the end of the second week. This network provides the fibroblasts with oxygen and nutrients so that they are able to synthesize collagen properly.

A subpopulation of fibroblasts become myo-fibroblasts. These specialized fibroblasts have the contractile properties of smooth muscle cells and exert a central pull on the wound edges, thereby decreasing the size of the wound. This process of wound contraction has usually been achieved by the third week. The rapid rise in tensile strength during this period parallels the increase in collagen content although the wound still has less than 15 per cent of its ultimate strength at this time (Madden, 1976; Madden and Peacock, 1971).

Management

The wound is now able to withstand the stress of gentle active movement. Protective splinting will need to be maintained in certain circumstances, e.g. following tendon repair. Pressure to scar is maintained during this period; however, as the wound is still thin and fragile, overzealous exercise and excessive pressure should be avoided. Oedema management may still be necessary and remains a priority until it is eliminated. Where significant oedema persists, the tissues of the hand are in a state of reduced nutrition and inelasticity where adhesion formation can readily ensue (Hunter and Mackin, 1995).

3. Remodelling or maturation phase

The remodelling phase lasts a minimum of 6 months but can continue for up to 2 years. At the beginning of this phase, the scar may be raised, red, thick and unyielding. With time, the scar will soften, becoming paler, flatter and more pliable. This phase sees a decrease in fibroplastic activity and a shutdown in mitotic activity. The wound gradually becomes stronger as the amount of collagen decreases although the tensile strength of scar tissue is never more than 80 per cent of that of uninjured skin.

Scar remodelling is characterized by the rapid, ongoing production of new collagen and the removal of old collagen. The initial gel-like collagen with its randomly arranged fibrils and low tensile strength is gradually replaced with stronger and more highly organized collagen.

Management

It is during this stage of high collagen turnover (2 to 4 months postinjury) that clinical treatment methods can exert their greatest influence and hence optimize functional outcome. The process of scar remodelling is favourably influenced by the application of low-load forces that are applied at the appropriate time (Arem and Madden, 1976). This is achieved through splinting and pressure therapy.

Tools of treatment

Hand injuries or conditions invariably present with one or all of the following:

1. Pain.
2. Swelling.
3. Scar.
4. Stiffness.

The therapist has a variety of treatment tools at his or her disposal. Choice of treatment modalities will be influenced by the professional and clinical background of the therapist (i.e. occupational or physiotherapist), possible budget restraints and the requests of the referring surgeon.

The therapist

At the patient's initial session, the most important treatment tool is the therapist. It is at this time that the patient's trust and confidence will need to be engendered for therapy to proceed. This means that the patient must be handled with great care, both physically and psychologically. Assessment and treatment should be as pain-free as possible and instructions to the patient should be clear and few in number. Ideally, they should be written down and accompanied by easily understood line drawings for home reference.

There are occasions when family involvement will be required. These situations include: the complex hand injury, children, the frail elderly, where there is a language difficulty or where patients feel unable to cope with the aftercare programme. The therapist also plays an important role in providing emotional support and as a motivator. This is especially important following major trauma where a protracted rehabilitation process is anticipated.

Clinical aspects of treatment

The therapy programme will need to address at least one, if not all, of the following:

1. Wound care.
2. Pain management.
3. Oedema control.
4. Exercise.
5. Scar management.
6. Splinting.
7. Desensitization.
8. Sensibility assessment/retraining.
9. Nerve gliding exercises.
10. Functional activity.
11. Psychological support.

Specific treatment modalities

The treatment modalities described below are those that the author believes are indispensable to hand therapy practice. These are also modalities that the patient is able to use away from the formal therapy environment. The home programme is a vital part of the rehabilitation process. Self-reliance is an essential component of psychological and emotional well-being and is encouraged as soon as the patient is ready. Patient education is therefore an important element in management.

Because many of these modalities can frequently address several clinical problems simultaneously, this section describes each modality in turn rather than management of individual clinical problems, i.e. pain, swelling, stiffness or scar. While this list is by no means exhaustive, it will address most of the clinical problems that the therapist is likely to encounter.

1. Exercise

Movement, both passive and active, is important in:

1. Maintaining joint mobility.
2. Maintaining the gliding function of tendons and nerves.
3. Helping eliminate oedema through compression and relaxation of the hand's tissues.

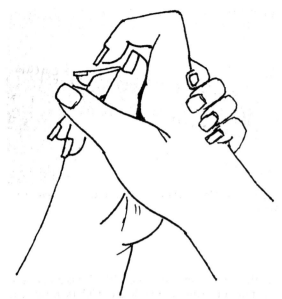

Figure 2.1. Unless contraindicated, active exercise is commenced as soon as possible after injury or surgery. Stabilized joint movement promotes differential tendon glide and generally results in a greater arc of motion, particularly when oedema is present.

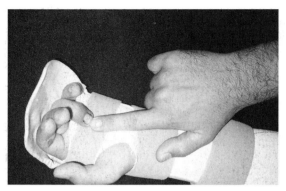

Figure 2.2. Passive movements need to be performed with great care to avoid exacerbating or causing pain and inflammation. For this reason, it is best if patients are taught to carry out their own exercises.

Active exercise

Active movement, where not contraindicated (e.g. following tendon repair), is begun as soon as possible after injury or surgery. In the early phase of therapy, exercise sessions are brief and frequent but should not exacerbate pain, inflammation or swelling. Movements should, however, be carried out in a systematic fashion that does not merely involve wriggling the fingers. Patients are given a specific number of repetitions to perform, e.g. 5 to 10 movements every 1 or 2 hours.

Where possible, movements should be performed in a stabilized manner so that differential tendon glide can occur. This entails stabilizing the joint or joints proximal to the joint being moved (Fig. 2.1). Individual stabilized movements generally result in a greater arc of motion than do composite joint movements. This is especially true where dorsal hand skin is 'taken up' by oedema with the effect of limiting global flexion.

Passive exercise

Passive exercises should be performed with great care so that again, pain, inflammation and oedema are not exacerbated. This is particularly important in the acute phase of management. For this reason, passive exercises are best performed by the patient who will generally perform them to a pain-free limit. Where appropriate, passive exercise should precede active exercise so that the muscle-tendon unit does not have to overcome the resistance of a stiff joint. This is particularly important in tendon rehabilitation (Fig. 2.2).

2. Coban wrap

Coban wrap is a thin, self-adherent elastic wrap that comes in various widths, the narrowest of which is 25 mm. Its sheerness makes it particularly suitable for use with fingers as it does not impede interphalangeal joint motion. Coban wrap should be replaced if it becomes wet. It is used:

(a) To control oedema

Acute digital oedema is effectively managed with the narrowest Coban wrap. A single layer is applied in a distal to proximal direction with negligible tension, so that the Coban is lain, rather than stretched onto the finger (Fig. 2.3). Patient instruction in its application is most important so that circulation is not compromised. Signs that the wrap has been applied too tightly include: (i) discoloration of the fingertip, (ii) throbbing and (iii) numbness or paraesthesia. These signs will usually manifest themselves within minutes of application and indicate that the wrap needs to be removed and reapplied.

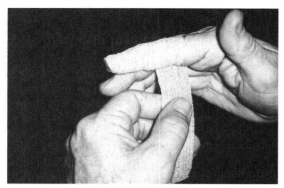

Figure 2.3. Acute digital oedema is most effectively managed with the narrowest Coban wrap (i.e. 25-mm-width). A single layer is applied in a distal to proximal direction under negligible tension.

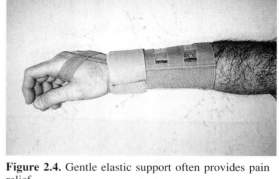

Figure 2.4. Gentle elastic support often provides pain relief.

Coban wrap is ideal for holding dressings in place as its minimal bulk allows greater ease of interphalangeal joint movement. Wider sizes of wrap can be applied to the dorsum of the hand; however, more economical alternatives include the use of an elastic crepe bandage or a single or double layer of appropriately sized tubular stockinette.

(b) To help prevent a PIP joint flexion deformity

The anatomy of the PIP joint favours flexion. The normal resting position of this joint is between 30 to 40 degrees (Bowers, 1987) and because oedema is more comfortably accommodated in this flexed position, a flexion deformity can quickly ensue. The gentle elastic tension of Coban wrap not only helps eliminate oedema but also exerts a mild extension force in the acute phase of treatment (e.g. after phalangeal fracture or Zone II flexor tendon repair).

(c) To help manage scar

The intimate contact that Coban wrap has with the skin makes it ideal for early pressure therapy over digital scar. The skin tolerates this wrap very well and it is relatively easy to remove and replace.

(d) To relieve pain

Patients frequently report pain relief when some form of gentle elastic support is applied to the area in question, e.g. an elastic wrist brace to support a painful wrist (Fig. 2.4). The PIP joint is a common location of pain in the hand. Coban wrap can facilitate increased interphalangeal joint range of movement through its pain-relieving effect.

3. Splinting

Hand splinting is an integral part of therapy during each phase of healing. Its initial role of protection and support is gradually supplanted by its corrective role in overcoming soft tissue and joint contracture, both of which can be the consequence of significant injury.

Types of splint

Splints can be categorized in a number of ways, i.e. static or dynamic, supportive or corrective, rigid or soft, volar or dorsal and forearm-, hand- or finger-based. A static splint has no moving components, unlike a dynamic splint which applies force through rubber bands or coils. Static splints are generally used to provide support and protection; however, they can behave dynamically when the splint is applied at the maximum range of joint movement or maximum soft tissue stretch. This is referred to as serial casting or splinting.

Splints can be used to optimize function by positioning the wrist and/or fingers when muscle power is absent (e.g. the radial nerve palsy splint that facilitates the reciprocal tenodesis effect) (Fig. 2.5) or to prevent joint and soft tissue contracture by controlling deformity and restoring balance in nerve lesions, e.g. the static 'spaghetti' splint for correction of ulnar 'claw' deformity

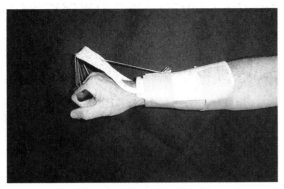

Figure 2.5. This forearm-based radial palsy splint restores the reciprocal tendosesis action of wrist extension-finger flexion and wrist flexion-finger extension.

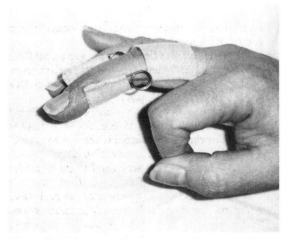

Figure 2.6. The dynamic hand-based Capener splint is manufactured from piano wire, thermoplastic material and adhesive moleskin. This splint is effective for overcoming PIP joint flexion deformities of 35 degrees or less.

(see Figure 5.14). The Capener splint is an example of a finger-based dynamic splint. This splint has a corrective function in overcoming PIP flexion deformities in the range of 15 to 35 degrees (Fig. 2.6). It is fashioned from piano wire, thermoplastic material and moleskin (see Colditz, 1995).

Splinting for tissue remodelling

Where exercise and soft tissue techniques prove insufficient in restoring joint and soft tissue mobility, corrective splinting is mandatory in achieving optimum functional results. Splinting is 'the only available therapeutic modality that applies controlled gentle forces to soft tissues for sufficient lengths of time to induce tissue remodelling without causing detrimental microscopic disruption of cellular structures' (Fess and McCollum, 1998).

The remodelling process cannot be achieved unless this gentle force is maintained over a period of weeks (and sometimes months). The tissue must be held under tension that is higher than its resting tension and must be applied continuously if permanent elongation of skin and other soft tissues is to occur (Bell-Krotoski and Figarola, 1995). Also, the viscous property of connective tissue must be subjected to a load of adequate intensity (Cyr and Ross, 1998). Forces ranging from 100 to 300 g are recommended for correcting contractures of the small joints of the hand (Brand, 1995).

It is preferable to err on the side of caution when splinting is begun so that tissue response can be monitored for any sign of swelling or inflammation. When the desired result has been achieved, intermittent splinting should be maintained throughout the remodelling phase until the tendency for relapse has been overcome. The timeframe for this will vary from patient to patient. A minimum of 6 months is recommended; however, patients should be encouraged to persevere for 12 to 18 months where the tendency for recidivism is high.

Principles of splinting

1. Prior to splint application, the patient will need to be educated in relation to the splint's purpose, application and wearing regimen (Fess, 1995). To maximize patient compliance, the splint should be simple in design, be easy to don and doff, be free of pressure areas and be as cosmetically pleasing as possible.
2. The splint should provide the minimum possible pressure so that the tissues of the hand can tolerate prolonged wear where necessary. This is best achieved by covering a larger area. Likewise, straps should be sufficiently wide and be angled to the contour of the forearm, hand or digit so that shear forces are avoided (Wilton, 1997). Slings used in dynamic splints need to pull at precisely 90 degrees if shear forces to the digit are to be avoided (Fig. 2.7).
3. The static portion of a dynamic splint should cover a sufficient area to ensure stability so that

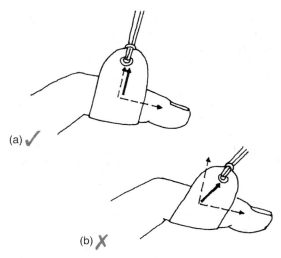

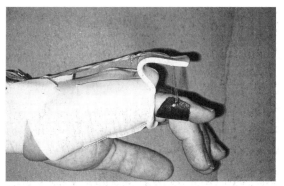

Figure 2.9. The joint proximal to the joint being mobilized will need to be well stabilized so that the corrective force that is applied remains constant. In the case of this dynamic outrigger to the PIP joint, the MCP joint has been stabilized in extension.

Figure 2.7. (a) When applying dynamic traction, the line of pull should be at a right angle to the axis of the skeletal segment being moved. (b) Where the line of pull is not at 90 degrees, a shear stress to the digit or hand segment will occur.

migration or rotation does not occur when forces are applied.

4. During flexion, the fingers converge toward the scaphoid bone. When applying a flexion force to the digit, the line of pull should follow this natural orientation (Fig. 2.8).
5. The joint proximal to the joint being mobilized needs to be well stabilized, e.g. the MCP joint is stabilized when an outrigger is applied to correct a PIP joint flexion deformity (Fig. 2.9).
6. Tolerance to splinting will need to be carefully assessed during the first few days. Skin is checked for signs of pressure areas or excessive sweating which may lead to skin maceration. Corrective splints are removed regularly throughout the day so that active movement and function can be maintained.

Soft splinting

Soft splinting refers to the use of soft materials such as neoprene (Clark, 1997), lycra, bandages (for flexion bandaging) or taping (e.g. Microfoam). These materials can address the following clinical problems:

1. Provide support and warmth to a painful joint.
2. Help to eliminate oedema.
3. Flatten scar that is raised or hypertrophic.
4. Exert a gentle corrective force to stiff or contracted joints (Figs 2.10 and 2.11).
5. Protect areas of hypersensitivity due to scar or a neuroma.

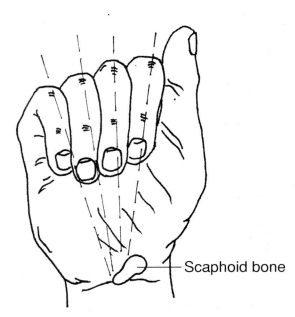

Figure 2.8. During flexion, the fingers converge towards the scaphoid bone. When applying a flexion force to the digit, this natural orientation will need to be accommodated.

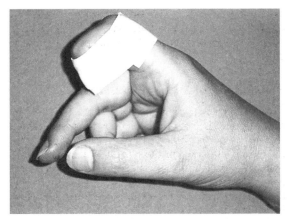

Figure 2.10. Microfoam (3M) tape makes an excellent interphalangeal joint flexion strap. It is soft, flexible and lightly adhesive.

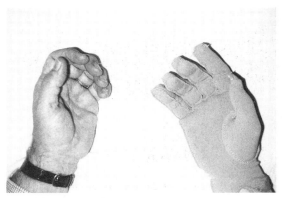

Figure 2.12. The 'extension force' of a lycra glove becomes apparent when a gloved and ungloved hand are compared.

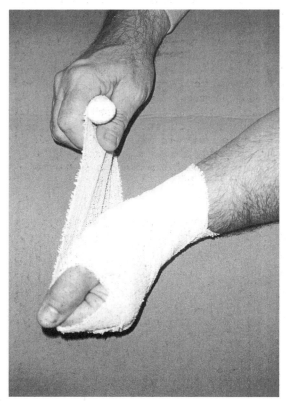

Figure 2.11. A crepe bandage (minimum 10 cm width) makes an excellent flexion wrap. Its effectiveness is augmented when the hand is immersed in warm water.

The extension force that a lycra glove can transmit through the interphalangeal joints is readily observed when a gloved and ungloved hand are compared. While lycra gloves are usually fitted to overcome hand oedema, in the painful hand they can be effectively used as a first-stage 'extension splint' prior to the fitting of a 'hard' splint (Fig. 2.12).

Advantages of neoprene and lycra

1. A high comfort factor ensures excellent patient compliance. For example, a neoprene finger-stall to correct a PIP joint flexion deformity can be worn around the clock without interfering with function because the fingertip can remain free and the stall allows virtually unrestricted flexion range (Fig. 2.13).
2. These fabrics are relatively economical.
3. The risk of pressure areas is negligible (particularly with neoprene).
4. Fingerstalls and wrist/thumb wraps can be manufactured in minutes. An older style sewing machine can be purchased at low cost and is able to handle thicker fabrics with ease. The sewing machine has become almost as integral to splinting as have the heating pan and heat gun.
5. Soft splints can be used in combination with thermoplastic splinting.

Because neoprene does not fray when cut, it is a very practical material to work with. To avoid pressure on the skin, seams are worn to the outside.

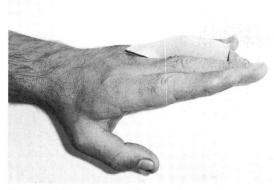

Figure 2.13. A neoprene fingerstall can make an effective 'extension' splint when continuously worn. It also helps eliminate digital oedema and provides effective compression to scar.

While not entirely cosmetic, the effectiveness of these stalls and garments far outweighs this slight disadvantage and is of little concern to most patients.

4. Silicone gel for scar management

Clinical studies have demonstrated the benefits of silicone gel sheeting in the prevention and treatment of hypertrophic scar (Katz, 1992). Cica-care gel is ideal for use on the hand because, although this product is quite expensive, hand scars are generally quite small. This, combined with the fact that the gel can be reused for some weeks, makes it a cost effective treatment (Fig. 2.14).

The gel is worn at least 12 h each day for 6 to 8 weeks in 'non-aggressive' scar and for up to 6 months where scar is hypertrophic or keloid. It is thought that hydration of the scar may reduce collagen deposition by decreasing capillary activity (Davey et al., 1991). Although the gel is adhesive, it should be held in place with tubular stockinette or paper tape (e.g. Micropore) so that it is not lost.

The gel is applied to skin that is healed, clean and dry. All traces of massage cream or oil should be removed prior to its application. Initial wearing times should be restricted to about 4 h so skin reaction to the gel can be assessed. Reaction is rare and will usually manifest as small red dots that resemble a heat rash. The skin should be 'aired' regularly to avoid maceration and the gel washed in a mild soapy solution at least once a day. Care should be taken to rinse and dry the gel thoroughly before reapplication.

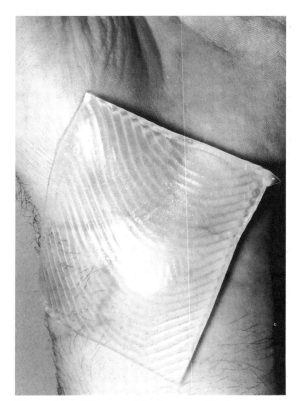

Figure 2.14. Silicone gel is the most effective treatment for raised or hypertrophic scarring. It can be used on its own or worn beneath a compression glove, tubular stockinette or Coban.

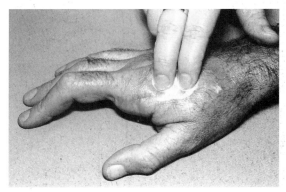

Figure 2.15. Gentle scar massage and percussion exercises initiate the desensitization process. The patient is encouraged to 'handle' the scar regularly throughout the day.

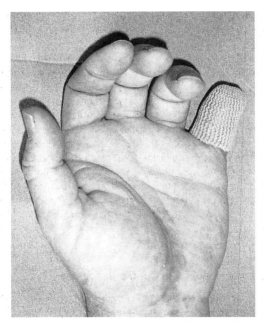

Figure 2.16. Silicone-lined fingerstalls help soften scar, shape the stump and provide protection.

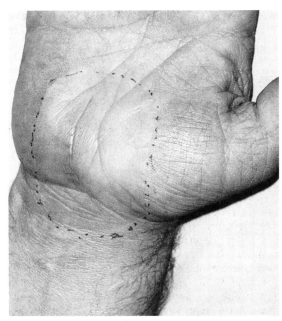

Figure 2.17. Opsite Flexifix is used to provide relief of pain and hypersensitivity related to scar, neuroma, fingertip injury, stumps, causalgia related to CRPS and paraesthesia associated with nerve regeneration. In this case it is used to lessen scar hypersensitivity following open carpal tunnel decompression.

Apart from impacting on the scar's topography and rendering it flat, pale and supple, the gel decreases pain and acts as a 'shock absorber' to sudden contact. The author believes that use of silicone gel is superior to scar massage as a treatment to soften scar. Scar massage is beneficial as a desensitizing exercise and to moisturize the skin.

5. Opsite Flexifix

Opsite dressings have been known to relieve pain when applied to wounds (Neal et al., 1981). Pain relief from contact of Opsite on unbroken skin in diabetic patients with painful neuropathy was anecdotal until a study was undertaken by the Diabetic Department of King's College Hospital in London (Foster et al., 1994). This study concluded that Opsite reduced pain in a significant number of patients with painful diabetic neuropathy.

While the pain of neuropathy results from a disease process rather than direct nerve or soft tissue injury, the types of symptoms commonly described by hand patients are common to both pathologies, i.e. shooting (lancinating), burning (causalgia), pins and needles (paraesthesia) or the extreme contact discomfort known as allodynia (Boscheinen-Morrin and Shannon, 2000).

Rationale

It is thought that Opsite may act in a similar way to transcutaneous electrical nerve stimulation (TENS) in that continuous contact of the film with the skin may stimulate the large, light touch A-beta afferent fibres and, in doing so, inhibit the nociceptive activity of the small A-delta and C-fibres, i.e. Melzack and Wall's 'gate-control theory' (Melzack, 1973).

The product

Opsite Flexifix (i.e. 'Opsite on a roll') is a non-sterile version of the original Opsite dressing. Opsite is an adherent polyurethane film which is waterproof and permeable to oxygen and water vapour. It is used in conjunction with 'Skin-Prep' wipes which enhance adhesion of the film to the skin. Opsite Flexifix is available in two widths. The narrower version, i.e. 5 cm roll, is more suitable for use on the hand.

Indications for use

1. Fingertip injuries.
2. Amputation stumps.
3. Causalgic pain associated with chronic regional pain syndrome.
4. Neuroma.
5. Scar hypersensitivity.
6. Paraesthesia associated with nerve regeneration.

The film is applied as soon as skin has healed. It is well tolerated by the skin and often remains in place for several days before needing to be replaced. Its sheerness and elasticity mean that movement is not affected when the film is applied across joints. Its use after fingertip injuries is ideal as sensibility is not impeded. The finest monofilament can be detected through the film. Opsite can be used beneath silicone gel. Even when used on its own, Opsite has a positive influence on scar as it exerts a gentle compressive force.

6. Transcutaneous electrical nerve stimulation

The advantage of TENS over other forms of pain relieving treatment is that pain relief is ongoing and not therapy dependent. Sensory level stimulation, i.e. conventional TENS (high pulse rate and narrow pulse width) delivers a therapeutic current to the cutaneous sensory afferent fibres. The amplitude is monitored to ensure that no muscle contraction is evident (Fig. 2.18).

Electrodes should only be used on skin that is intact and has sensation. TENS is not used by patients with pacemakers. Electrode placement is often a matter of experimentation. Electrodes should not be placed immediately over the painful area. The electrode is placed over the peripheral nerve, proximal to the site of pain or injury or on either side of the area (i.e. proximal and distal). The current is increased gradually until the patient perceives a comfortable level of stimulation which is continued for 30–60 min at a time. A carry-over effect is often experienced for several hours. The unit is reapplied when this effect begins to diminish.

Some specific indications for use

1. Causalgic (burning) pain associated with chronic regional pain syndrome (Types 1 and 2).
2. Neuritis following surgery or injury, e.g. irritation of the superficial branch of the radial nerve after surgery for Colles' fracture or decompression of the first dorsal compartment for de Quervain's syndrome.

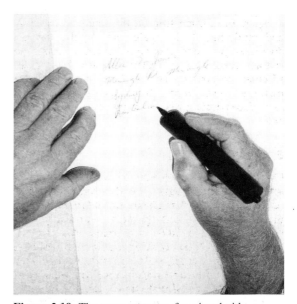

Figure 2.19. The most common functional aid involves the enlargement of handles. This is achieved easily and economically with different sizes of insulation tubing.

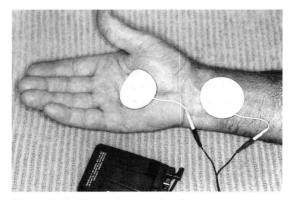

Figure 2.18. Transcutaneous electrical nerve stimulation can be particularly effective in managing neuritis that can follow surgical procedures, causalgia associated with CRPS or neuroma pain.

3. Hypersensitivity following carpal tunnel decompression.
4. Neuroma.

It is important that patients do not over-exercise or overuse the hand during periods of pain relief. Exercises and activity are carried out slowly and gently and response is monitored prior to upgrading the therapy programme.

7. Aids to daily living

Until a functional range of motion has been restored, it can be helpful to modify the small handles of everyday utensils. This is achieved simply and economically with insulation tubing usually referred to as 'Handitube' (Fig. 2.19). This product is available from most major hardware stores. For patients with ongoing functional limitation and/or weakness, many excellent labour-saving devices are now available from department stores.

References

Alvarez, O. (1989). Moist environment in healing: Matching dressing to wounds. *Wounds*, **2**, 59.

Arem, A. and Madden, J. (1976). Effect of stress on healing wounds: Intermittent noncyclical tension. *J. Surg. Res.*, **20**, 93.

Bell-Krotoski, J. A. and Figarola, J. H. (1995). Biomechanics of soft tissue growth and remodeling with plaster casting. *J. Hand Ther.*, **8(2)**, 131–7.

Boscheinen-Morrin, J. and Shannon, J. (2000). Opsite Flexifix: An effective adjunct in the management of pain and hypersensitivity in the hand. *Aust. J. Occ. Ther.*, (submitted September, 2000).

Bowers, W. H. (1987). The anatomy of the interphalangeal joints. In *The Interphalangeal Joints* (W. H. Bowers, ed.) pp. 13–20, J. B. Lippincott.

Brand, P. W. (1995). The forces of dynamic splinting: Ten questions before applying a dynamic splint to the hand. In *Rehabilitation of the Hand: Surgery and Therapy* (J. M. Hunter, E. J. Mackin and A. D. Callahan, eds) pp. 1581–7, Mosby.

Brand, P. W. (1998). Mechanical factors in joint stiffness and tissue growth. *J. Hand Ther.*, **8(2)**, 91–6.

Clark, E. N. (1997). A preliminary investigation of the neoprene tube finger extension splint. *J. Hand Ther.*, **10(3)**, 213–21.

Colditz, J. C. (1995). Spring-wire extension splinting for the proximal interphalangeal joint. In *Rehabilitation of the Hand: Surgery and Therapy* (J. M. Hunter, E. J. Mackin and A. D. Callahan, eds) pp. 1617–29, Mosby.

Cyr, L. M. and Ross, R. G. (1998). How controlled stress affects healing tissues. *J. Hand Ther.*, **11(2)**, 125–30.

Davey, R. B., Wallis, K. A. and Bowering, K. (1991). Adhesive contact media: an update on graft fixation and burn scar management. *Burns*, **17**, 313–9.

Fess, E. E. (1995). Principles and methods of splinting for mobilization of joints. In *Rehabilitation of the Hand: Surgery and Therapy* (J. M. Hunter, E. J. Mackin and A. D. Callahan, eds) pp. 1589–1598, Mosby.

Fess, E. E. and McCollum, M. (1998). The influence of splinting on healing tissues. *J. Hand Ther.*, **11(2)**, 157–61.

Foster, A. V. M., Eaton, C., McConville, D. O. and Edmonds, M. E. (1994). Application of Opsite Film: A new and effective treatment of painful diabetic neuropathy. *Diab. Med.*, **11**, 768–772.

Hardy, M. A. (1986). Preserving function in the inflamed and acutely injured hand. In *Hand Rehabilitation* (C. A. Moran, ed.) pp. 1–15, Churchill Livingstone.

Hugo, N. (1977) General aspects and healing of skin. In *Biological Aspects of Reconstructive Surgery* (D. Kernahan and L. Vistness, eds) p. 339, Little, Brown and Co.

Hunt, T. K. and Hussain, Z. (1992). Wound microenvironment. In *Wound Healing: Biochemical and Clinical Aspects* (I. K. Cohen, R. F. Diegelmann and W. J. Lindblad, eds) pp. 274–81, W. B. Saunders.

Hunter, J. M. and Mackin, E. J. (1995). Edema: Techniques of evaluation and management. In *Rehabilitation of the Hand: Surgery and Therapy* (J. M. Hunter, E. J. Mackin and A. D. Callahan, eds) pp. 77–85, Mosby.

Katz, B. E. (1992). Silastic gel sheeting is found to be effective in scar therapy. *Cosm. Derm.*, **1**, 3.

Madden, J. W. (1976). Wound healing: The biological basis of hand surgery. *Clin. Plast. Surg.*, **3(1)**, 3.

Madden, J. W. and Peacock, E. E. (1971). Studies on the biology of collagen during wound healing. III: Dynamic metabolism of scar collagen and remodeling of dermal wounds. *Ann. Surg.*, **174**, 511.

Melzack, R. (1973). *The Puzzle of Pain*. Penguin Education.

Neal, D. E., Whalley, P. C., Flowers, M. W. and Wilson, D. H. (1981). The effects of an adherent polyurethane film and conventional absorbent dressing in patients with small partial thickness burns. *Br. J. Clin. Pract.*, **35**, 7–8.

Peacock, E. E. (1984). *Wound Repair*. W. B. Saunders.

Smith, K. L. (1995). Wound care for the hand patient. In *Rehabilitation of the Hand: Surgery and Therapy* (J. M. Hunter, E. J. Mackin and A. D. Callahan, eds) pp. 237–50, Mosby.

Wilton, J. C. (1997). Biomechanical principles of design, fabrication and application. In *Hand Splinting: Principles of Design and Application*. pp. 22–42, W. B. Saunders.

Witte, C. and Witte, M. (1971). Significance of protein in edema fluid. *Lymphology*. **4**, 29.

3

Flexor tendons

Function and anatomy

The function of tendons is to attach muscle to bone and transmit muscle action across joints. Tendons are dense connective tissues composed largely of collagen. Individual bundles of collagen are covered by endotenon. The surface of the tendon is covered by a fine fibrous outer layer called the epitenon. A thin visceral layer, the paratenon, covers the flexor tendon fascicles in the hand (Strickland, 1999).

The orderly parallel arrangement of the collagen fibres equips tendons to cope with the high unidirectional tensile loads to which they are subjected during activity. While tendons are strong enough to sustain these tensile forces, they are also sufficiently flexible to curve around bone and joint surfaces and to deflect beneath the retinacular pulley system during finger flexion.

Like bone, tendon remodels in response to the mechanical demands placed upon it. Collagen organization is significantly disturbed in the absence of tension. Tendon becomes stronger when subjected to increased stress and weaker when stress is reduced (Hitchcock et al., 1987).

The flexor sheath and pulley system

The flexor tendon sheath is composed of synovial and retinacular components. The synovial component is a tube which is sealed at both ends where its visceral and parietal layers merge (Doyle, 1989). In the index, middle and ring fingers, the synovial portion of the sheath begins at the metacarpal neck and extends as far as the DIP joint. The synovial

sheath of the little finger and thumb extends proximally to the wrist (Fig. 3.1).

The synovial portion of the sheath is overlain with a series of pulleys of varying configurations, i.e. transverse, annular and cruciform. These pulleys represent the retinacular portion of the flexor sheath. The palmar aponeurosis (PA) pulley is formed from the transverse fibres of the palmar aponeurosis and was described by Manske and

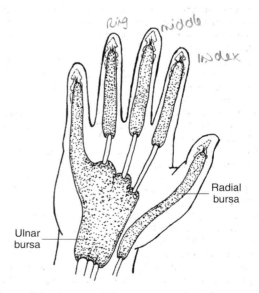

Figure 3.1. The synovial component of the flexor tendon sheath. The synovial sheaths of the thumb and little finger extend proximally to the wrist. The sheath of the thumb is the radial bursa; the sheath of the little finger is the ulnar bursa.

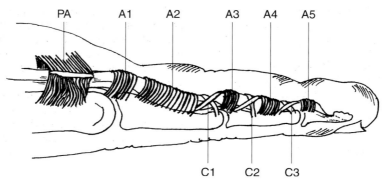

Figure 3.2. The pulley system overlying the synovial component of the flexor tendon sheath represents the retinacular portion of the sheath. These pulleys hold the tendon in close proximity to the skeleton and facilitate efficient joint motion with minimal tendon excursion. They also prevent the tendon from bowstringing. They are comprised of: the palmar aponeurosis pulley (PA), five rigid annular pulleys and three thin, pliable cruciate pulleys.

Lesker (1983). The cruciate pulleys, i.e. C1, C2 and C3, are thin and pliable and collapse to facilitate full digital flexion (Fig. 3.2).

In the digits there are five rigid annular (or ring-shaped) pulleys, i.e. A1, A2, A3, A4 and A5. The thumb has one oblique and two annular pulleys. These pulleys keep the flexor tendons in close proximity to the phalanges and joints. This facilitates efficient joint motion with minimal tendon excursion via a short moment arm. Biomechanically, the most important of the pulleys are the A2 and A4 pulleys. Their absence results in bowstringing of the tendon and an increase in moment arm. This, in turn, results in loss of digital movement (Fig. 3.3).

Tendon nutrition

Flexor tendons receive nutrition from vascular and synovial sources. Vascular perfusion outside the digital sheath is via mesotendineal vessels. Within the digital sheath, blood supply is provided segmentally via the long and short vincula (Armenta and Lehrman, 1980) (Fig. 3.4).

Synovial fluid diffusion delivers nutrients to the tendon and retinacular system via a process known as imbibition. This is a pumping mechanism where fluid is forced into the interstices of the tendon as the digit is being flexed and extended. This process is especially important to the two avascular structures where friction and gliding take place, i.e.

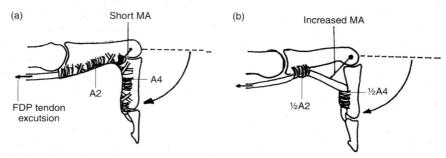

Figure 3.3. (a) The A2 and A4 pulleys are the most important biomechanically. The close proximity of the flexor tendons to the phalanges and joints creates a short moment arm and efficient motion. (b) When portions of these two pulleys are resected, an increase in moment arm occurs and greater tendon excursion is required to move the joint through the same arc of motion. Note the bowstringing of the unrestrained tendon. (Reproduced from Strickland, J. W. Flexor tendons-acute injuries. 1999. In *Green's Operative Hand Surgery* (D. P. Green, R. N. Hotchkiss and W. C. Pederson, eds) p. 1855, Churchill Livingstone, with permission.)

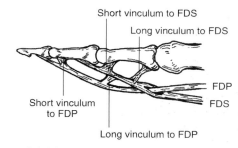

Figure 3.4. Vincular blood supply of the flexor tendons.

the palmar aspect of the flexor tendons and the inner aspect of the pulleys.

As well as providing nutrition to the retinacular system and tendon, synovial fluid acts as a lubricating agent to facilitate the tendon turning a corner.

Tendon healing

Tendons have both an intrinsic and extrinsic ability to heal. For some time it was thought that the tendon itself was not involved in the healing process but rather that union could only be achieved via invasion of the healing area by paratendinous tissues. Research, however, has shown that the tendon does play an active role in the repair process (Lundborg et al., 1985).

Extrinsic healing is characterized by adhesions between the tendon and its surrounding tissues. Intrinsic healing results in fewer and less dense adhesions. The healing process involves three distinct but overlapping phases:

1. Inflammatory – this phase lasts 3 to 5 days. The strength of the repair at this stage is tenuous and is imparted almost entirely by the suture.
2. Fibroblastic – this phase begins at about the fifth day and lasts for 3 to 6 weeks. This is the collagen-producing phase during which strength increases rapidly.
3. Remodelling – this maturation phase continues for 6 to 9 months. This phase sees a continuation of collagen synthesis and longitudinal orientation of fibroblast and collagen fibres. The repair continues to gain strength during this period.

Timing of tendon repair

Although no longer considered an emergency, primary tendon repair should ideally be performed within the first few days of injury to yield the best possible outcome (Gelberman et al., 1991b). While delayed primary repair can be performed up to 3 weeks, some deterioration of tendon ends and shortening of the muscle-tendon unit becomes inevitable.

Contraindications for primary repair include: severe injury to multiple tissues, wound contamination or significant skin loss over the flexor surface. Tendon reconstruction can be managed at a later date by two-stage tendon grafting.

Incisions for surgical exposure

The wound sustained by the injury is usually transverse or oblique and will need to be extended to allow tendon repair. The skin laceration is usually extended to produce a zigzag approach using points and lines of minimal tension to reduce scar. Alternatively, a midaxial approach is made on either side of the finger and then connected to the original laceration. Retrieval of retracted tendon ends is achieved by proximal-to-distal milking of the tendons or with the help of a silastic cannula.

Tendon repair technique

Repair of the tendon is performed as atraumatically as possible. Wherever the tendon surface is punctured by forceps, a site of potential tendon adhesion is created (Potenza, 1964). Both flexor tendons should be repaired. The tendon sheath is repaired whenever possible so that the potential for synovial fluid nutrition is restored. The repaired sheath also serves as a barrier to the formation of extrinsic adhesions.

The divided tendon ends are repaired as accurately as possible without tension and with the least interruption to the blood supply. A core suture with 3–0 or 4–0 nonabsorbable thread is used. A peripheral circumferential epitendinous suture (continuous 6–0 monofilament) is used in addition to the core suture (Mashadi and Amis, 1992). This suture provides significant increase in the strength of the repair and reduction of gapping between the tendon ends.

Biomechanical studies suggest that strength of the repair is proportional to the number of suture strands that cross the repair site (Wagner et al., 1994). Four-strand core sutures are about twice as strong as two-strand methods and six-strand sutures, three times stronger. When using a two-strand method, the repair is considered somewhat vulnerable for the first three weeks after surgery.

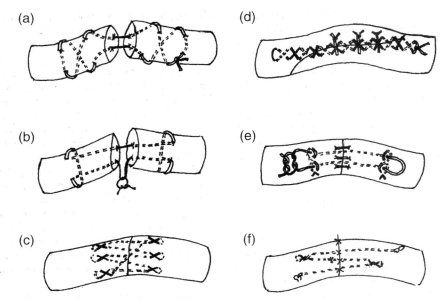

Figure 3.5. Various techniques of repairing flexor tendons. (a) Bunnell, (b) modified Kessler, (c) single cross-grasp six-strand (Sandow and McMahon), (d) Becker (bevel technique), (e) Tsuge (f) six-strand using three suture pairs (Lim and Tsai).

Four- and six-strand repairs however, are considered capable of withstanding light unresisted active motion in the presence of full passive interphalangeal flexion (Fig. 3.5).

Zones of tendon repair

Zone I is the most distal zone where only the flexor digitorum profundus (FDP) can be divided. This zone is distal to flexor digitorum superficialis (FDS) insertion.

Zone II has been called 'no man's land' because of previously poor results following repair in this zone which extends from the A1 pulley to the FDS insertion and where both flexor tendons travel in the flexor sheath.

Historical note

The term 'no man's land' originated in the Middle Ages and refers to an area outside the northern wall of London where the bodies of criminals were displayed following hanging, beheading or impaling. This served as a warning to others. When gallows were eventually built inside the city proper and the surrounding land was settled and fields were cultivated, the former execution grounds were claimed by no man.

Much later, around 1900, the phrase became part of military parlance.

Zone III extends from the A1 pulley to the distal edge of the transverse carpal ligament. This is the zone of lumbrical origin. Injuries to this zone have

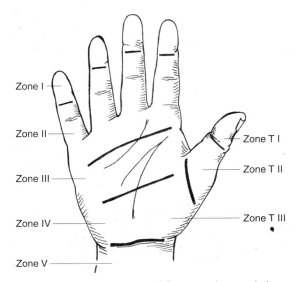

Figure 3.6. The five zones of flexor tendon repair in the digits and three zones of repair for flexor pollicis longus.

good results because it lies beyond the flexor sheath and restrictive adhesions are less likely.

Zone IV is the carpal tunnel and tendon laceration in this zone can be accompanied by injury to the median and/or ulnar nerves. Tendon injuries are less common in this zone due to the relative protection afforded by the transverse carpal ligament and bony architecture of the tunnel. Zone V covers the distal portion of the forearm extending from the musculotendinous junction to the proximal edge of the transverse carpal ligament (Fig. 3.6).

Early application of stress following tendon repair

Early application of stress to a healing tendon can biologically affect scar remodelling. Gelberman and others (1980, 1990, 1991a) have demonstrated the following benefits associated with early passive mobilization of tendons in dogs:

1. Faster recovery of tensile strength.
2. Fewer adhesions.
3. Improved tendon excursion.
4. Minimal deformation at the tendon site.

Historical perspective of postoperative flexor tendon management

A number of postoperative programmes have evolved over the past few decades. Their aim has been to provide differential gliding of the FDS and FDP tendons within the constricted space of Zone II. Passive flexion of the interphalangeal joints pushes the tendon proximally while active or passive interphalangeal joint extension pushes the tendon distally.

These programmes have undergone and continue to undergo modifications in response to increased knowledge of tendon nutrition and biology. The original controlled motion protocol was devised by Kleinert (1967). This involved rubber band traction which maintained the digit in a flexed posture while allowing active extension of the interphalangeal joints against the tension of the rubber band.

Duran and Houser (1975) later devised a protocol which maintains the interphalangeal joints in extension. Passive flexion exercises are performed individually at the DIP joint, then the PIP joint and finally at all three finger joints simultaneously (Fig. 3.7).

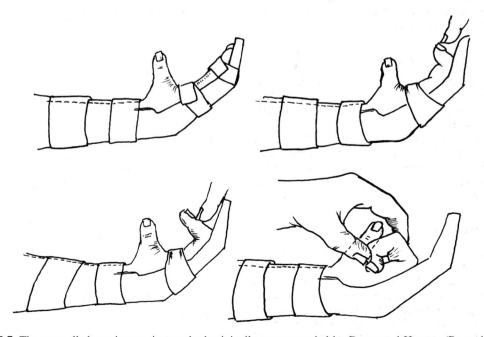

Figure 3.7. The controlled passive motion method originally recommended by Duran and Houser. (Reproduced from Strickland, J. W. Flexor tendons-acute injuries. 1999. In *Green's Operative Hand Surgery* (D. P. Green, R. N. Hotchkiss and W. C. Pederson, eds) p. 1866, Churchill Livingstone, with permission.)

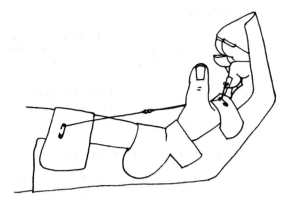

Figure 3.8. The incorporation of a distal palmar pulley provides maximum passive flexion of both interphalangeal joints. This splint was designed by Linwood Thomas, OTR, for the 'Washington regimen'. (Reproduced from Chow, J., Thomas, L., Dovelle, S., et al. 1987. A combined regimen of controlled motion following flexor tendon repair in 'no man's land'. *Plast. Reconstr. Surg.*, 79, 447–453, with permission.)

McGrouther and Ahmed (1981) concluded that it was necessary to passively flex the joints distal to the repair in order to achieve glide of the repair site. Subsequent studies suggest that aftercare programmes should aim at maximum passive flexion of both interphalangeal joints. This has resulted in the incorporation of a distal palmar pulley (Brooke Army splint) such as that seen in the 'Washington regimen' described by Chow and associates (1990). The addition of a distal palmar pulley (which has also been incorporated into the Kleinert regimen) maintains both interphalangeal joints at almost full flexion when the hand is at rest (Fig. 3.8).

Controlled active motion protocols

The last decade has seen the evolution of controlled active motion protocols (Bainbridge, 1994). The introduction of four- and six-strand repair methods together with strong peripheral epitendinous suturing have facilitated 'place and hold' flexion of the interphalangeal joints using

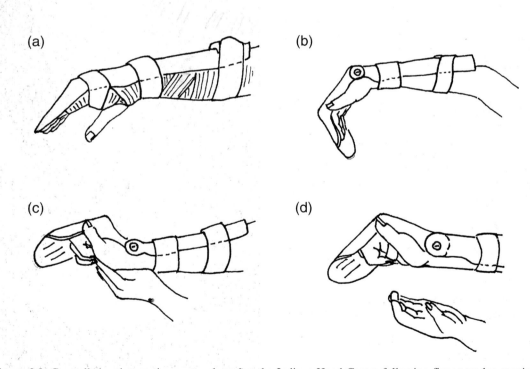

Figure 3.9. Controlled active motion protocol used at the Indiana Hand Centre following flexor tendon repair. (a) The conventional dorsal splint is worn most of the time. (b–d) The dynamic tenodesis splint, which is only used for the first four weeks after surgery, is used on an hourly basis following passive finger flexion exercises within the static splint. (Reproduced from Strickland, J. W. Flexor tendons-acute injuries. 1999. In *Green's Operative Hand Surgery* (D. P. Green, R. N. Hotchkiss and W. C. Pederson, eds) p. 1867, Churchill Livingstone, with permission.)

minimal muscle-tendon tension. Some surgeons believe that a two-strand repair with strong peripheral epitendinous suturing can withstand early active motion. The 'place and hold' manoeuvre is performed with the wrist in 45 degrees of extension and maximum MCP joint flexion as this position produces the least tension on the repaired tendon (Savage, 1988) (Fig. 3.9).

The dynamic tenodesis splint developed at the Mayo clinic by Cooney et al. (1989) uses this principle. Controlled active motion protocols have been described by Allen et al. (1987), Cullen et al. (1989), Small et al. (1989), Strickland (1993), Cannon (1993), Evans and Thompson (1993) and Silverskjoeld and May (1994).

Choice of treatment programme

Many hand centres have developed their own programme using different aspects of one or all of the described methods. The programme used with our patients for Zone II is outlined below and exemplifies a combined approach.

Each surgeon has particular views and preferences and the therapy regimen will obviously be influenced by these. The level of experience of the treating therapist will also dictate treatment choice. Other important factors influencing the choice of programme include:

1. The presence of associated injuries, e.g. damage to the neurovascular bundle or fractures.
2. The age of the patient.
3. The patient's ability and/or willingness to comply with the programme.
4. The type of scar produced by the patient, i.e. supple tissue with minimal reaction or dense, fibrous tissue.

Aims of therapy

Regardless of which particular programme is used, the following aims are inherent in achieving a favourable outcome:

1. Control of postoperative oedema.
2. Regaining flexibility of the interphalangeal joints.
3. Prevention of PIP joint flexion deformity.
4. Scar management.

Postoperative management

The protocol outlined below refers specifically to repair of the flexor tendon(s) in Zone II. It is, however, applicable to all zones.

Splint position

Following surgery the hand is placed in a dorsal plaster which maintains the wrist in neutral extension and the MCP joints in maximum flexion, this usually ranging from 75 to 90 degrees. Elevation of the limb is maintained. Shoulder and elbow exercises are begun within a day of surgery and repeated every 1 to 2 hours.

Exercise protocol from 3rd to 24th day

On the 3rd or 4th postoperative day, when the inflammatory response has usually settled, the plaster is replaced with a thermoplastic splint which maintains the hand in the same position as the postoperative plaster. Gentle passive interphalangeal (IP) joint flexion exercises are commenced and performed only within comfortable limits (Fig. 3.10). The index finger can be placed behind

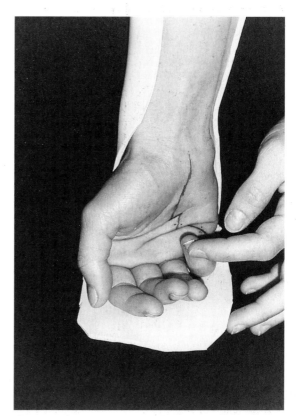

Figure 3.10. Gentle passive interphalangeal joint flexion exercises are commenced on the 3rd postoperative day. They are performed within comfortable limits and repeated on an hourly basis.

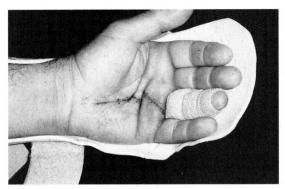

Figure 3.11. Active intrinsic interphalangeal joint extension exercises are also repeated on an hourly basis. The patient should aim to extend to the limit of the splint, i.e. full IP joint extension. This is often not possible during the first few days due to oedema and wound discomfort.

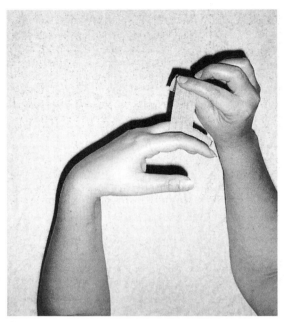

Figure 3.12. Coban wrap compression (25 mm) provides an excellent means of eliminating digital oedema. It is applied more easily when the hand is removed from the splint and allowed to fall into maximum wrist flexion so that the fingers relax in extension where they will fall slightly apart. One layer of Coban applied under negligible tension is sufficient.

the proximal phalanx of the involved digit while the thumb places light pressure to the fingernail so that both IP joints are flexed simultaneously. If there has been associated digital nerve repair, the exercises are carried out with even greater care as hypersensitivity at the repair site is common.

Each passive flexion manoeuvre is held for a short period (i.e. 30–60 s) and is followed by active intrinsic IP joint extension (Fig. 3.11). Both passive flexion and active intrinsic extension are usually limited at this early stage by digital oedema and discomfort; however, when performed on an hourly basis with 5 to 10 repetitions, improvement is usually seen quite rapidly within the first few days. Under ideal circumstances, full passive IP joint flexion and full active IP joint extension should be achieved by the end of the second postoperative week. Sutures are removed at this time.

Active movement of flexor digitorum superficialis (FDS)

If FDS is intact, it can be exercised by trapping the DIP joints of the unaffected fingers in extension and then gently flexing the PIP joint of the affected digit. This helps maintain glide of the uninjured FDS tendon. This exercise is only performed when the IP joints can be passively flexed to full range with ease.

Note: If a controlled active motion protocol has been requested, the author uses the 'tenodesis manoeuvre' described in the 'Day 24 to end of week 6' section. This manoeuvre is performed two

to three times every 4 h during these first $3\frac{1}{2}$ weeks and is held for 1 to 2 seconds only with minimal effort. It is only performed when full passive flexion has been achieved.

Resolution of digital oedema

Digital swelling often subsides significantly following the commencement of the exercise routine. Application of a single layer of Coban (25 mm) will effectively address residual oedema. This is applied carefully by the therapist in a distal to proximal direction and can be done so more easily if the hand is removed from the splint, the elbow rested on the table and the wrist allowed to fall into maximum flexion; this will result in the fingers assuming a relaxed position of IP joint extension which will see the digits slightly separate (Fig. 3.12).

Flexion deformity of the PIP joint

The combination of hourly active intrinsic IP joint extension exercises and Coban is usually sufficient

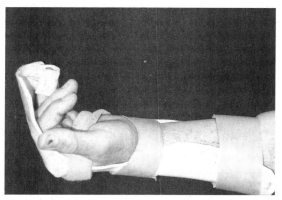

Figure 3.13. Patients who heal with dense scarring often have an increased propensity toward PIP flexion deformity. This can be managed with a sling that applies negligible extension force to the digit. Where necessary, the sling is used during sleep. During the day, the sling is removed hourly to perform passive IP joint flexion exercises.

to prevent the development of a PIP joint flexion deformity. Where a deformity has developed, it can be addressed with a small thermoplastic splint that is applied to the dorsum of the joint in a position of slight correction; this is gradually modified until full correction has been achieved.

Alternatively, a soft 'sling' is placed on the volar aspect of the middle phalanx. Nylon thread is then attached to holes punched through the sides of the sling. The nylon is then threaded through a hole made in the splint and attached to a hook on the outside of the splint. The tension applied by the sling should be negligible and the line of pull should be at right angles to the middle phalanx. The sling is removed for hourly passive IP joint flexion exercises and intrinsic IP joint extension exercises (Fig. 3.13).

Scar management

Following suture removal, the hand is bathed in warm soapy water to cleanse the skin. To protect the tendon repair, the wrist should be passively held in maximum flexion range. If passive IP joint flexion range is still restricted, the warmth of the water will make passive flexion exercises easier. Also, the fingers can be gently bandaged into flexion prior to immersion in the water. This will necessitate the wrist being brought into neutral extension while the fingers are passively held in the flexed position.

Gentle oil massage is performed to soften the scar and to begin the desensitization process. The latter is especially important where the digital nerve repair has also been performed. Massage can be performed out of the splint by the therapist; however, when the patient is performing the massage, it is safer to keep the hand within the splint and undo the distal splint strap if necessary. Finger pressure should be very light during the first few sessions until increased pressure can be tolerated. If hypersensitivity is problematic enough to interfere with the exercise programme, covering the area with Opsite Flexifix will often reduce hyperaesthesia significantly.

If Coban wrap is not already being used for swelling control, it should be added to the programme for its effectiveness in providing gentle compression to scar. Unless scar is particularly dense, this modality can be used alone. Where raised, dense scar restricts passive flexion or is painful to touch, silicone gel is used under the Coban during the night and intermittently throughout the day.

Day 24 to end of week 6

At $3\frac{1}{2}$ weeks gentle active flexion exercises are begun. Prior to the commencement of active exercise, the patient must first 'warm up' with passive flexion exercises. Active flexion is only begun if the patient is able to passively flex both IP joints to near-normal flexion range with ease. The last few degrees of passive flexion can sometimes be restricted by dense scarring or residual oedema.

As a tendon glides, it meets a certain degree of normal resistance from surrounding tissues. This is referred to as 'drag'. Following injury and surgery, this resistance is significantly increased due to swelling, sutures and healing scar. The newly repaired tendon must not, therefore, be subjected to the added stress of overcoming joint stiffness when active movement is commenced.

Every 2 h the hand is removed from the splint and rested comfortably on the table in neutral wrist extension. From their flexed position, the MCP joints are actively extended to within 20 or 30 degrees of full extension and gently supported. This more extended MCP joint position will help accommodate extrinsic finger flexion.

With the wrist in neutral and the MCP joints supported in 20 to 30 degrees of flexion, the patient is asked to actively extend the IP joints to their maximum range as they have been doing in the

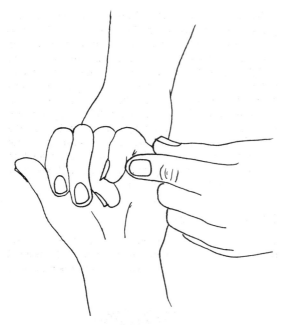

Figure 3.14. Gentle combined active IP joint flexion (i.e. both IP joints simultaneously) is practised second-hourly with 5–10 repetitions at each session. Active range of motion is usually still quite limited at this early stage. Patients who demonstrate significant active range with ease are 'held back' because they tend to be at greater risk of rupture due to minimal scar formation.

splint. When maximum IP joint extension range is reached, the patient is then asked to actively flex both IP joints simultaneously with minimal effort (Fig. 3.14). This position is gently held for several seconds before the exercise is repeated. Five to ten repetitions are performed. These early attempts may yield 30 or 40 degrees of PIP joint flexion and 20 or 30 degrees DIP flexion. From the 4th week onward, the MCP joints can be increasingly extended during IP joint flexion exercises to better facilitate flexor tendon pull-through.

Patients who demonstrate marked active flexion range are considered at greater risk of rupture due to minimal scar formation. These patients are protected for a longer period. This means that the commencement of active movement is delayed by another week and protective splinting is continued for 1 to 2 weeks longer. When active movement is then initiated, it can be done so with the less-stressful tenodesis manoeuvre described below. Resisted use of the hand will also be delayed by several weeks.

Tenodesis manoeuvre

If active flexion range is minimal or where the risk of rupture is considered greater, the patient should be shown 'place and hold' exercises as it takes less force to maintain an already flexed finger in the flexed position than it does to actively bring the finger into flexion from the extended position. This manoeuvre involves passively flexing the fingers, allowing the wrist to extend to 40 to 45 degrees and then removing the passive support and asking the patient to maintain the flexed finger position with minimal active muscle-tendon tension (Fig. 3.15(a)). Savage (1988) has shown that this position produces the least tension on the repaired tendon during active movement. This position is held for 3 to 5 seconds. The wrist is then brought

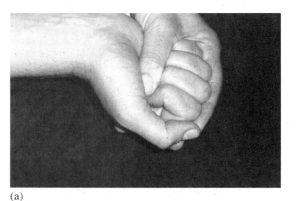

(a)

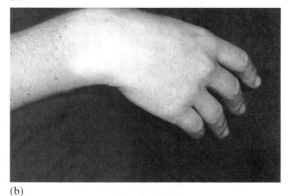

(b)

Figure 3.15. (a) The first part of the 'tenodesis manoeuvre' involves passively flexing the fingers and allowing the wrist to assume a position of 45 degrees extension. Passive support is then removed and the patient is asked to maintain the flexed position with minimal active muscle-tendon tension. (b) The wrist is then brought forward into flexion while the fingers gently extend.

forward into flexion while the fingers gently extend, i.e. the tenodesis effect. This manoeuvre is repeated 5 to 10 times second hourly (Fig. 3.15(b)).

The patient may find it helpful to perform their active exercises in both of the described ways.

Weeks 6 to 8

The splint is discarded at the end of the 6th postoperative week unless the nature of the scar indicates that extended protection is necessary. The hand can be used for light daily functional activities that are minimally resistive. The light (sustained) squeezing of a soft bath sponge in warm water is a suitable exercise at this stage. Patients whose work does not involve heavy manual activity usually return to work at this stage.

Residual flexion deformity of the PIP joint is addressed with a neoprene fingerstall (Fig. 3.16). If adhesions are affecting tendon glide, the use of an MCP joint blocking splint will facilitate pull-through of the extrinsic flexors (Fig. 3.17).

During activity, the injured finger can be buddy-taped to an adjacent finger with Microfoam tape if limitation of active flexion range makes gripping objects difficult. Small handles such as cutlery or razor can be temporarily built up with insulation tubing (i.e. Bradflex). Light-grade exercise putty can be added to the programme by the 7th week. Putty squeezing should be carried out in a slow and sustained manner and the patient should take care not to over-exercise. Three or four short sessions (5 min) each day are sufficient as the patient should also be engaging the hand in regular activity (Fig. 3.18).

Repair in Zones III, IV and V is often accompanied by tethering of the tendon to skin and surrounding tissues and some shortening of the muscle-tendon unit. This can be addressed with serial volar splints which exert a gentle corrective extension force and are worn at night and intermittently throughout the day. Occasionally soft tissue tightness is quite marked. This may warrant the use of a dynamic outrigger. Regardless of the splinting method used, the tension applied should be low and the correction should be gradual to avoid rupturing the repair. The patient should feel a gentle stretching sensation that is not painful.

Week 8 onwards

Gentle resistance is added to active flexion exercises and activity can be upgraded. Stabilized exercises are continued; however, they need not be

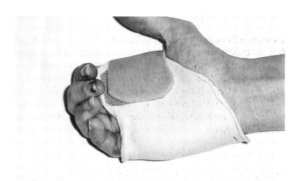

Figure 3.17. An MCP joint blocking splint will facilitate pull-through of the extrinsic flexor tendons.

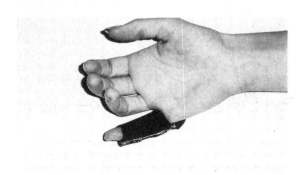

Figure 3.16. Unresolved flexion deformities of the PIP joint are managed with a neoprene fingerstall from the 6th week onward.

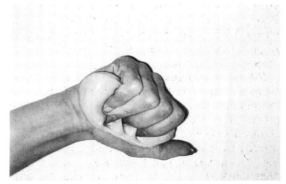

Figure 3.18. Light-grade exercise putty is added to the programme by the 7th week.

repeated as frequently. Return of function is more of a priority at this stage in rehabilitation and patients are encouraged to perform domestic or mechanical tasks as part of their therapy programme if they have not yet returned to work.

Patients whose work is heavily resistive do not return to work in their normal capacity until the end of the 12th week. This period is extended for a further 2 weeks where scar formation has been minimal.

Note: Many patients make steady gains in active flexion range during the first 3 to 4 postoperative months. Patients who heal with dense scar frequently show slower progress. Final range of active motion may not be achieved for some months following cessation of formal therapy. Patients are therefore encouraged to persevere with their exercise/activity programme.

Flexor pollicis longus (FPL) repair

Splint position

The splint is applied to the dorsum of the forearm and hand, with the wrist in neutral or very slight flexion. The thumb is held in slight palmar abduction with the MCP in 30 degrees of flexion and the IP joint in neutral extension. The tip of the thumb should be in line with the middle finger (Fig. 3.19).

Exercise protocol

The exercise protocol is the same as for repair of a digital flexor tendon. Some patients find it difficult to isolate FPL function and tend to overuse the intrinsic thenar muscles when active exercises are

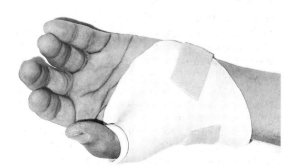

Figure 3.20. To avoid compensatory movements by the intrinsic thumb muscles during IP joint flexion exercises, a blocking splint is used to isolate the action of flexor pollicis longus.

begun. This tendency can be overcome with an MCP blocking splint which will restrict movement to the long thumb flexor. This can be applied between the 4th and 5th week (Fig. 3.20).

Tenolysis

Any injury or operation that interferes with the smooth gliding surface of the tendon system predisposes the tendon to becoming adherent to adjacent tissues, i.e. skin, retinacular ligament and bone. A tenolysis procedure aims to free the tendon from its adhesions and restore its glide. Secondary joint changes (capsule or ligament fibrosis) may also need correction.

Tenolysis is indicated only when comprehensive therapy measures, used over a period of at least 3 to 6 months following injury or surgery, have failed to restore a functional range of movement (Fetrow, 1967 and Baker et al., 1996). Patient selection is most important as strong motivation and full co-operation are required in the postoperative phase. Patients are advised that two-stage tendon reconstruction may be necessary if the tendon motor and/or flexor pulley system prove inadequate.

Technique

The procedure is performed under local anaesthetic using a zig-zag incision. By using this type of anaesthesia, the patient is awake and able to participate so that the surgeon is able to carry out just enough dissection and freeing.

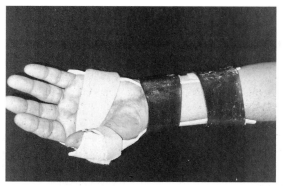

Figure 3.19. Postoperative splint used following repair of flexor pollicis longus.

Postoperative management

The immediate postoperative exercise regimen will vary from patient to patient and will be determined by the integrity of the freed tendon. Poor quality tendons have a greater risk of rupture and should be exercised with some caution. Tendons deemed to be in good condition can be exercised more vigorously. Discussion with the attending surgeon is therefore essential.

The first postoperative week is the most important (Schneider and Berger-Feldscher, 1995). The aim of therapy is to reproduce the range of movement that was achieved during surgery, before adhesions have an opportunity to become re-established. The exercise regimen should be sufficient to promote maximum tendon glide without causing an inflammatory response or increasing oedema.

Splint

The hand can be rested in the position of safe immobilization, i.e. wrist comfortable extension, MCP joints in flexion and the IP joints in extension.

Oedema and pain control

The hand is maintained in elevation between exercise sessions and ice packs are used every 3 to 4 hours prior to exercise during the first 2 to 3 days to reduce swelling and discomfort. The immediate postoperative dressing may require de-bulking to ensure effectiveness of the ice pack and to facilitate exercise. Care is taken to keep the wound dry and sterile. Coban wrap can be applied over the dressing to help control swelling. A single layer is sufficient and should not interfere with exercise.

Appropriate pain relief should be provided prior to active exercise which is commenced on the day of surgery.

Exercise protocol (days 0 to 7)

Where the tendon is deemed to be at risk of rupture, only 'place and hold' exercises are performed during the first week as they require less tensile loading. The fingers are passively flexed to a comfortable range by the therapist or the patient's uninvolved hand. This position of passive flexion is held for a short period (i.e. 30–60 s) after which time the supporting hand is removed and the patient is asked to maintain the

position with minimal active muscle-tendon tension for several seconds. The digits are then gently extended (actively) and the manoeuvre is repeated another 3 to 5 times. The exercise session is repeated every 3 to 4 hours during the first day and on an hourly basis from then on. Each session should see a slight increase in flexion range.

Where tendon integrity is considered sound, gentle active unstabilized finger exercises are begun. They should be preceded by passive exercises so that the tendon does not have to overcome the resistance of stiffened joints. The exercises are repeated 3 to 4 times on the first day and hourly thereafter. Response to exercise is monitored on an individual basis and the programme is modified accordingly.

Optimizing tendon glide

To promote optimal tendon glide, the fingers are exercised in a variety of ways:

1. MCP joints are flexed with the IP joints held in extension, i.e. intrinsic plus position.
2. A hook grip is made, i.e. the IP joints are flexed while the MCP joints are maintained in extension.
3. Composite flexion involves simultaneous flexion of all three finger joints. To provide further differentiation, the fist can be 'flat', i.e. with the DIP joints in extension while the MCP and PIP joints are flexed, or 'tucked', i.e. with the DIP joints flexed.

Wrist movements are also practised at each exercise session together with movements of the shoulder, elbow and forearm.

Days 7 to 14

Stabilized (or blocking) exercises are added to the active exercise programme for 'low risk' tendons. Splints that block the MCP joints in extension and provide more effective pull-through of the flexor tendon can be used by the end of the 2nd week. For more vulnerable tendons, 'place and hold' exercises are replaced with gentle unstabilized composite flexion exercises from a position of digital extension. Stabilized exercise for 'at risk' tendons is delayed until the 3rd postoperative week.

Sutures are removed around the 14th day and oil massage and scar management are begun. Silicone gel can be used beneath Coban or a silicone-lined finger sleeve can be worn. Light gripping activities can be commenced at this time.

Day 14 onwards

Scar management, active exercise and light activity are continued. Resisted exercise and activity can commence at week 6 and full resistance can be tolerated after the 8th week.

Two-stage tendon reconstruction

Where tendon glide has been compromised by injury and/or surgery and tenolysis has been unsuccessful, tendon function can be restored with a two-stage procedure (Hunter et al., 1995).

Patient selection for two-stage tendon reconstruction is even more important than for tenolysis because it requires two surgical procedures and a personal and economic commitment to a protracted aftercare programme.

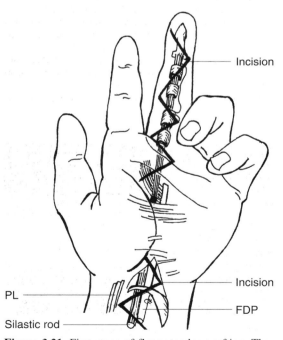

Figure 3.21. First stage of flexor tendon grafting. The implant (silastic rod) is attached to the distal tendon stump and then threaded along the digit and through the carpal tunnel to lie freely, proximal to the wrist.

Preoperative requirements

1. Full or near-normal passive flexion of the IP joints.
2. Full or near-normal digital extension.
3. Soft supple tissues.

Stage 1

The scarred tendon is resected and replaced with a silastic implant or 'rod'. The implant is attached to the distal tendon stump. It is then threaded along the digit and through the carpal tunnel to lie freely proximal to the wrist. The muscle motor is anchored to the adjacent muscle-tendon unit if FDP is involved or to the flexor retinaculum if FPL is involved. Annular pulleys are reconstructed over the implant around which a fibrous pseudosheath forms during the next 8 to 10 weeks (Fig. 3.21).

This first stage may also involve scar correction, nerve repair/graft or capsulotomy to improve joint range of motion.

Postoperative aims

1. To regain passive flexion and active extension range.
2. To soften scar tissue and restore soft tissue mobility in preparation for the second stage.
3. To maintain mobility of all upper limb joints.
4. To encourage use of the hand in suitable light activity.

Postoperative management

Days 1 to 14

For the first 2 weeks the hand is rested on a volar splint with the wrist in slight extension or neutral and the fingers close to neutral extension. No passive IP joint flexion exercises or active wrist movements are performed during this time. The purpose of rest is to safeguard against silicone synovitis which has been associated with early postoperative exercise. Adjacent finger joints can be gently exercised. Oedema is managed with elevation and ice packs.

Day 14 onwards

The sutures are removed and massage to scar is commenced. Gentle passive IP joint flexion and active IP extension exercises are begun. Gentle active wrist movement is also carried out. These exercises are to be performed slowly and carefully and within the limits of pain. Over-vigorous exercise can easily result in synovitis. Short sessions (1–2 min duration) every 2 h are sufficient during the first week of exercise. Early signs of synovitis can include:

1. Sudden increased swelling along the volar aspect of the finger.
2. Pain at rest or during passive flexion.
3. Loss of passive range.
4. Swelling over the proximal end of the implant, i.e. at the wrist.

Normal residual digital oedema is treated with a single layer of Coban wrap. Scar is managed with a silicone-lined fingerstall which is worn throughout the night and intermittently during the day. Silicone gel is used over palmar scar.

If the patient has difficulty in regaining flexion range, the hand is bandaged gently into flexion several times a day or a digital flexion strap is used; only the gentlest of pressure is used during these manoeuvres. The patient is not permitted to engage the hand in heavy activity while the implant is present. To encourage flexibility of the affected digit, it is buddy-strapped to an adjacent digit during light activity and exercise (Fig. 3.22).

Stage 2

The second stage of reconstruction is usually performed 8 weeks after the first and involves removal of the implant and a tendon graft. Incisions are made over the distal and proximal juncture sites. The tendon graft (palmaris longus, plantaris or a long toe extensor) is harvested and sutured to the proximal end of the implant. It is then pulled through the new tendon bed.

At the distal juncture, the tendon is drawn into the bone with monofilament stainless steel or a nonabsorbable suture. The wire is tied over a button on the dorsum of the fingernail; this remains in place for a minimum of 6 weeks. The proximal end of the graft is attached to the motor tendon with a Pulvertaft end-weave technique.

Postoperative management

The aftercare regimen is as for primary repair with the proviso that the programme is carried out more cautiously. Because the grafted tendon has a more precarious blood supply, there is increased risk of rupture. For this reason, the various therapy 'milestones' are all delayed by approximately one week (Fig. 3.23).

References

Allen, B. N., Frykman, G. K., Unsell, R. S. and Wood, V. E. (1987). Ruptured flexor tendon tenorrhaphies in Zone II: repair and rehabilitation. *J. Hand Surg.,* **12A**, 18–21.

Armenta, E. and Lehrman, A. (1980). The vincula of the flexor tendons of the hand. *J. Hand Surg.,* **5**, 127–34.

Bainbridge, D. P., Robertson, C., Gillies, D. and Elliot, D. (1994). A comparison of postoperative mobilization of flexor tendon repairs with 'passive flexion-active extension' and 'controlled active motion techniques'. *J. Hand Surg.,* **19B**, 517–21.

Baker, M. K., Dunn, S. J., Tonkin, M. A. and Eakins, D. F. (1996). Flexor tenolysis: a worthwhile procedure in a select patient population. *Hand Surg.,* **1**, 131–40.

Cannon N. (1993). Post flexor tendon repair motion protocol. *Indiana Hand Center Newsletter,* **1**, 13.

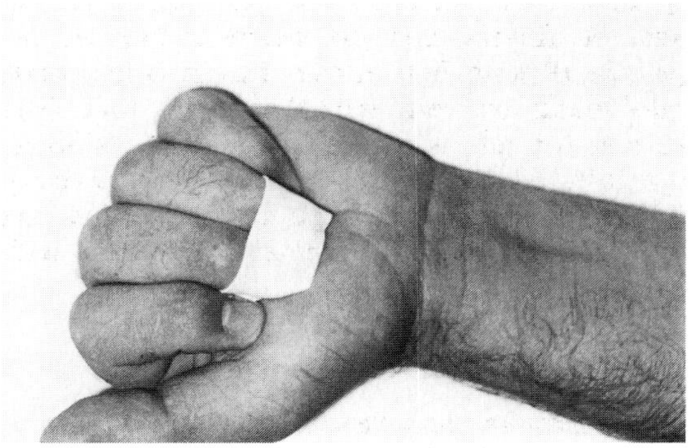

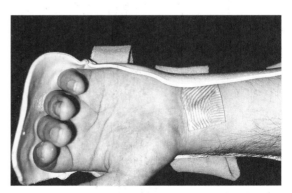

Figure 3.22. To maintain interphalangeal joint flexibility of the affected digit, it is 'buddy-strapped' to an adjacent digit during light activity. Microfoam tape makes an effective buddy-strap as it is soft, flexible and reusable.

Figure 3.23. The aftercare regimen following the second stage of reconstruction is as for primary repair; however, the various therapy milestones are delayed by 1 to 2 weeks. Note use of silicone gel to soften the wrist scar.

Chow, S. P., Stephens, M. M., Ngai, W. K., et al. (1990). A splint for controlled active motion after flexor tendon repair. Design, mechanical testing and preliminary clinical results. *J. Hand Surg.*, **15A**, 645–51.

Cooney, W. P., Lin, G. T. and An, K. T. (1989). Improved tendon excursion following flexor tendon repair. *J. Hand Surg.*, **2**, 102–6.

Cullen, K. W., Tolhurst, P., Lang, D. and Page, R. E. (1989). Flexor tendon repair in zone II followed by controlled active mobilization. *J. Hand Surg.*, **14B**, 392–5.

Doyle, J. R. (1989). Anatomy of the flexor tendon sheath and pulley system: a current review. *J. Hand Surg.*, **14A**, 349–51.

Duran, R. J. and Houser, R. G. (1975). Controlled passive motion following flexor tendon repair in zones II and III. In *AAOS Symposium on Tendon Surgery of the Hand*, pp. 105–14, Mosby.

Evans, R. B. and Thompson, D. E. (1993). The application of force to the healing tendon. *J. Hand Ther.*, **6**, 266–84.

Fetrow, K. O. (1967). Tenolysis in the hand and wrist. A clinical evaluation of two hundred and twenty flexor and extensor tenolyses. *J. Bone Joint Surg.*, **49A**, 667–85.

Gelberman, R. H., Khabie, V. and Cahill, J. C. (1991a). The revascularization of healing flexor tendons in the digital sheath: a vascular injection study in dogs. *J. Bone Joint Surg.*, **73A**, 868–81.

Gelberman, R. H., Menon, J., Gonsalves, M. and Akeson, W. H. (1980). The effects of mobilization on the vascularization of healing flexor tendons in dogs. *Clin. Orthop.*, **153**, 283–89.

Gelberman, R. H., Siegel, D. B., Savio, L., et al. (1991b). Healing of digital flexor tendons: importance of the interval from injury to repair. *J. Bone Joint Surg.*, **73A(1)**, 66.

Gelberman, R. H., Woo, S. L. Y., Amiel, D., et al. (1990). Influences of flexor sheath continuity and early motion on tendon healing in dogs. *J. Hand Surg.*, **15A**, 69–77.

Hitchcock, T. F., Light, T. R., Bunch, W. H., et al. (1987). The effect of immediate constrained digital motion on the strength of flexor tendon repairs in chickens. *J. Hand Surg.*, **12A**, 590–5.

Hunter, J. M, Taras, J. S., Mackin, E. J., et al. (1995). Staged flexor tendon reconstruction using passive and active tendon implants. In *Rehabilitation of the Hand: Surgery and Therapy* (J. M. Hunter, E. J. Mackin and A. D. Callahan, eds) pp. 477–514, Mosby.

Kleinert, H. E., Kutz, J. E., Ashbell, T. S. and Martinez, E. Primary repair of lacerated flexor tendons in 'no-man's land' (abstract). *J. Bone Joint Surg.*, **49A**, 577.

Lundborg, G., Rank, F. and Heinau, B. (1985). Intrinsic tendon healing: a new experimental model. *Scand. J. Plast. Reconstr. Surg.*, **19**, 113–7.

Manske, P. R. and Lesker, P. A. (1983). Palmar aponeurosis pulley. *J. Hand Surg.*, **8**, 259–63.

Mashadi, Z. B. and Amis, A. A. (1992). Strength of the suture in the epitenon and within the tendon fibres: development of stronger peripheral suture technique. *J. Hand Surg.*, **17B(2)**, 172.

McGrouther, D. A. and Ahmed, M. (1981). Flexor tendon excursions in 'no man's land. *Hand*, **13**, 129.

Potenza, A. D. (1964). Prevention of adhesions to healing digital flexor tendons. *J. A. M. A.*, **187**, 187–91.

Savage, R. (1988). The influence of wrist position on the minimum force required for active movement of the interphalangeal joints. *J. Hand Surg.*, **13B**, 262–8.

Schneider, L. H. and Berger-Feldscher, S. (1995). Tenolysis: Dynamic approach to surgery and therapy. In *Rehabilitation of the Hand: Surgery and Therapy* (J. M. Hunter, E. J. Mackin and A. D. Callahan, eds) pp. 463–75, Mosby.

Silverskjoeld, K. L. and May, E. J. (1994). Flexor tendon repair in zone II with a new suture technique and an early mobilization program combining passive and active motion. *J. Hand Surg.*, **19A**, 53–60.

Small, J. O., Brennen, M. D. and Colville, J. (1989). Early active mobilization following flexor tendon repair in zone 2. *J. Hand Surg.*, **14B**, 383–91.

Strickland, J. W. (1993). Flexor tendon repair: Indiana method. *Indiana Hand Center Newsletter*, **1**, 1.

Strickland, J. W. (1999). Flexor tendons-acute injuries. In *Green's Operative Hand Surgery* (D. P. Green, R. N. Hotchkiss and W. C. Pederson, eds) pp. 1851–97, Churchill Livingstone.

Wagner, W. F., Carroll, C., Strickland, J. W., et al. (1994). A biomechanical comparison of techniques of flexor tendon repair. *J. Hand Surg.*, **19A**, 979–83.

Further reading

Aoki, M., Kubota, H., Pruitt, D. L. and Manske, P. R. (1997). Biomechanical and histological characteristics of canine flexor repair using early postoperative mobilization. *J. Hand Surg.*, **22A**, 107–14.

Amadio, P. C., Jaeger, S. H. and Hunter, J. M. (1995). Nutritional aspects of tendon healing. In *Rehabilitation of the Hand: Surgery and Therapy.* (J. M. Hunter, E. J. Mackin and A. D. Callahan, eds) pp. 409–16, Mosby.

Callan, P. P. and Morrison, W. A. (1994). A new approach to flexor tendon repair. *J. Hand Surg.*, **19B**, 513–6.

Kleinert, H. E., Schepels, S. and Gill, T. (1981). Flexor tendon injuries. *Surg. Clin. North Am.* **61**, 267–86.

May, E. J., Silverskjoeld, K. L. and Sollerman, C. J. (1992). Controlled mobilization after flexor tendon repair in zone II: a prospective comparison of three methods. *J. Hand Surg.*, **17A**, 942–52.

Peck, F.H., Bucher, C. A., Watson, S. J. and Roe, A. E. (1996). An audit of flexor tendon injuries in zone II and its influence on management. *J. Hand Ther.*, **9**, 306–8.

Stewart, K. M. and van Strien, G. (1995). Postoperative management of flexor tendon injuries. In *Rehabilitation of the Hand: Surgery and Therapy.* (J. M. Hunter, E. J. Mackin and A. D. Callahan, eds) pp. 433–62, Mosby.

Strickland, J. W. (1989). Biologic rationale, clinical application, and results of early motion following flexor tendon repair. *J. Hand Ther.*, **2**, 71–8.

Taras, J. S., Gray, R. M. and Culp, R. W. (1994). Complications of flexor tendon injuries. *Hand Clin.*, **10**, 93–109.

Wehbe, M. A. (1987). Tendon gliding exercises. *Am. J. Occup. Ther.*, **41**, 164–7.

4

Extensor tendons

The dorsum of the hand has minimal subcutaneous tissue. This means that extensor tendons are vulnerable to injury due to their relatively superficial location. Extensor tendon injuries are generally regarded as less significant than those involving flexor tendons. Postinjury complications, however, are common and can include tendon adhesion, extensor lag and stiffness. Inadequate management can result in significant functional loss.

Anatomy

The extensor mechanism is characterized by numerous soft tissue attachments and interconnections (e.g. juncturae tendini). Unlike the flexor tendons which are surrounded by a synovial sheath, the extensor mechanism in the hand and fingers is covered by paratenon. The tendons in this region are broad and flat with a significant tendon-bone interface. The soft tissue attachments and the support of the paratenon ensure that retraction of the divided tendon is limited. As a result, many extensor tendon injuries, particularly those over the digits, can be treated conservatively with splinting (Fig. 4.1).

Over the dorsum of the wrist, the extensor tendons are considerably more substantial and are overlain by a wide fibrous band, the extensor retinaculum, the function of which is to prevent bowstringing of the tendons.

At this level the tendons are surrounded by a synovial sheath and held in place by five fibro-osseous tunnels (or compartments) and one fibrous tunnel, (the fifth dorsal compartment). These six compartments are separated by septa that arise from the retinaculum and insert onto the radius.

Dorsal compartments

The first compartment houses abductor pollicis longus and extensor pollicis brevis; the second, extensor carpi radialis longus and extensor carpi radialis brevis; the third, extensor pollicis longus; the fourth, extensor digitorum communis (EDC) and extensor indicis proprius; the fifth, extensor digiti minimi and the sixth, extensor carpi ulnaris. Just proximal to the MCP joints, the communis tendons are joined by fibrous interconnections known as juncturae tendini.

Dorsal hood of MCP joint

The dorsal hood of the finger MCP joints is a broad, fibrous structure combining fibres from the sagittal band, juncturae tendini and the extensor tendon. It serves to centre the EDC tendon, the primary extensor of the MCP joints.

Extensor mechanism of the digit

The extensor mechanism of the digit is a conjoint tendinous structure that is formed by the merging of the following structures (Fig. 4.2):

1. The extrinsic extensor digitorum communis (radial nerve).
2. The intrinsic volar and dorsal interossei (ulnar nerve).
3. The lumbrical muscles (ulnar and median nerves).

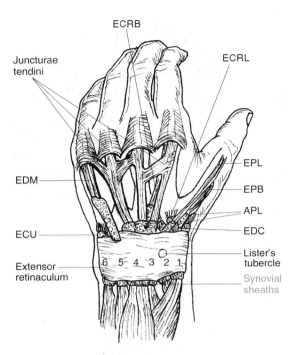

Figure 4.1. The extensor mechanism of the hand depicting the extensor tendons, the juncturae tendini, the extensor retinaculum, the six dorsal compartments and the synovial sheaths. (Copyright, Elizabeth Roselius, 1999. Reproduced from Doyle, J. R. Extensor tendons-acute injuries. In *Green's Operative Hand Surgery* (D. P. Green, R. N. Hotchkiss and W. C. Pederson, eds) p. 1951, Churchill Livingstone, with permission.)

1. Extensor digitorum communis

Distal to the MCP joint, the extensor tendon trifurcates into a central slip and two lateral slips. The central slip inserts into the base of the middle phalanx where it is joined by a medial band of oblique fibres from the lumbricals and interossei. The two lateral slips of the extensor tendon pass on either side of the PIP joint and join with the lateral bands of the intrinsic muscles to form the conjoined lateral bands. These unite distally as the terminal tendon and insert into the distal phalanx.

2. Intrinsic volar and dorsal interossei

The dorsal and volar interossei are separated from the lumbricals by the deep transverse metacarpal ligament. The interossei are the primary MCP joint flexors. They contribute to IP joint extension only when the MCP joints are simultaneously flexed.

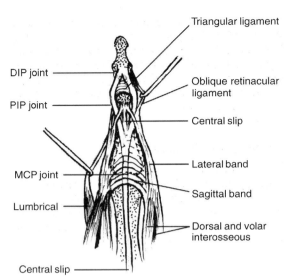

Figure 4.2. The extensor mechanism of the digits. (Copyright, Elizabeth Roselius, 1999. Reproduced from Doyle, J. R. Extensor tendons-acute injuries. In *Green's Operative Hand Surgery* (D. P. Green, R. N. Hotchkiss and W. C. Pederson, eds) p. 1953, Churchill Livingstone, with permission.)

3. The lumbricals

The lumbricals are unique in that they are the only muscles that arise from a flexor tendon and insert onto an extensor tendon. They arise from the tendon of flexor digitorum profundus and insert onto the radial lateral band of each finger. The lumbricals are the prime intrinsic interphalangeal joint extensors.

Retinacular ligaments

1. Transverse retinacular ligament

This ligament arises from the flexor sheath and volar plate at the PIP joint and passes to the lateral border of the conjoined lateral band. It prevents dorsal dislocation and bowstringing of the lateral bands during IP joint extension and serves to stabilize the extensor tendon over the PIP joint in the way that the sagittal band does at the MCP joint.

2. Oblique retinacular ligament (ORL)

The ORL passes from the flexor sheath of the proximal phalanx and joins the lateral margin of the terminal extensor tendon. Its course is volar to the axis of the PIP joint but dorsal to the axis of the DIP joint. The ORL is considered to be a retaining ligament that centralizes the tendon on the dorsum of the finger (Harris and Rutledge, 1972). It helps co-ordinate uniform flexion and extension of the PIP and DIP joints.

3. Triangular ligament

This ligament consists of a fascial layer between the conjoined lateral bands and the terminal tendon distal to the insertion of the central slip onto the middle phalanx. This ligament prevents excessive volar subluxation of the conjoined lateral bands on flexion of the PIP joint.

Zones of extensor tendon injury

The location of an extensor tendon injury will influence the type of treatment. It will also determine the deformity and functional impairment. The extensor mechanism can be injured from the fingertip (Zone I) to the middle or proximal forearm (Zone IX). The original classification by Kleinert and Verdan (1983) included eight zones in the digital extensor mechanism and five zones for the thumb. A ninth zone has now been added to the classification; it covers the muscular area over the middle and proximal forearm (Fig. 4.3).

Closed injuries

Closed injuries are best managed by splinting. Specific treatment regimens are discussed in each zone.

Surgery for open injuries

In the case of a tidy wound, primary extensor tendon repair is indicated as soon as possible after injury. This urgency is not as great as for flexor tendons because in Zones I to V the retinacular fibres and juncturae between the tendons prevent significant retraction of the proximal tendon end.

If the wound is dirty or contaminated, it should be debrided until satisfactory healing has occurred. A delayed primary procedure is then performed under optimal conditions, with additional skin coverage where required. The suture technique is modified according to the site of repair as the

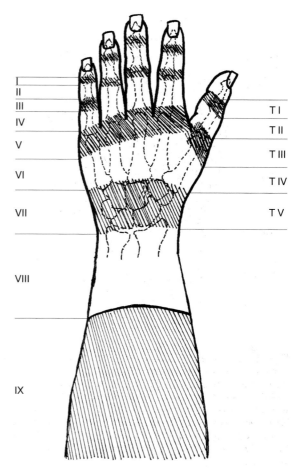

Figure 4.3. Zones of extensor tendon injury in the digits and thumb.

extensor mechanism becomes increasingly thin in its distal zones. A study by Newport et al. (1995) concluded that the Kleinert modification of the Bunnell suture and the modified Kessler technique provided the greatest strength and were able to tolerate controlled active motion protocols. The horizontal mattress suture is weaker than the weave sutures but is suitable for broad, flat tendons with longitudinal fibres.

In complex injuries involving loss of substance (particularly in Zone VI) or where there are fractures and joint injuries, soft tissue cover takes priority over tendon reconstruction. This should be by either a local or distant flap as skin grafts should not be applied over tendons (Fig. 4.4).

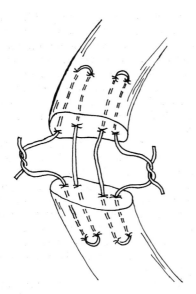

Figure 4.4. Technique for extensor tendon repair. The horizontal mattress suture is suitable for broad, flat tendons with longitudinal fibres.

Postoperative management: immobilization vs. early controlled mobilization

Repaired extensor tendons have traditionally been immobilized for a period of 3 to 4 weeks prior to the commencement of active movement. Because of the propensity toward tendon adhesion, treatment results were frequently disappointing. The introduction of controlled mobilization techniques in the management of extensor tendon injuries has led to improved results, particularly in the more challenging Zone III over the PIP joint.

Evans and Burkhalter (1986) reported their 6-year experience using controlled motion in the treatment of untidy extensor injuries. Their treatment protocol was developed using knowledge of extensor tendon excursion as reported by Bunnell (from Boyes, 1970), Elliot and McGrouther (1986) and Brand and Hollister (1993). The effectiveness of early dynamic splinting has been verified by Browne and Ribik (1989), Hung et al. (1990) and Saldana et al. (1991).

It has been suggested that 3–5 mm of tendon excursion (Duran and Houser, 1975 and Gelberman et al., 1986) is sufficient to promote glide and stimulate cellular activity without causing gapping or rupture of the repair. Evans and Burkhalter (1986) determined that 30 to 40 degrees of MCP joint motion effected 5 mm of extensor glide in Zones III, IV, V, VI and VII. In the case of extensor pollicis (EPL) repair, 60 degrees of IP joint flexion effected 5 mm of tendon excursion at Lister's tubercle with the wrist in neutral and the thumb MCP joint in extension.

The controlled passive and/or active mobilization protocol is only used with patients who are able to comply with the regimen. While the first few treatments are labour-intensive and time-consuming in terms of splint fabrication and patient education, the rate of progress and overall result far outweigh these initial commitments. Where patients being treated with immobilization are just commencing their active therapy programme at week 4, most patients being managed with the controlled mobilization protocol are nearing the end of formal therapy. It is our experience that patients involved in this protocol also benefit psychologically from early active participation.

The treatment programmes described below will include conservative management of closed injuries together with static and controlled mobilization protocols following surgical repair of extensor tendons. Discussion between surgeon and therapist is essential in determining the protocol most suitable for each patient.

Zones I and II

Interruption of the extensor mechanism over the DIP joint and the distal portion of the middle phalanx results in a flexion deformity of the joint, i.e. a mallet finger. The injury can be either closed or open. These injuries are frequently associated with a small avulsion fracture at the base of the distal phalanx where the tendon inserts (Fig. 4.5).

Conservative management of closed injury

Closed injuries are treated with a dorsal or volar splint which maintains the DIP joint in extension for a period of 6 to 8 weeks. The position of the DIP joint in the splint needs to be critically evaluated as even slight flexion at the joint will cause attenuation of the tendon callus and a resultant extensor lag. Correct positioning within the splint is best maintained with taping rather than strapping (Fig. 4.6).

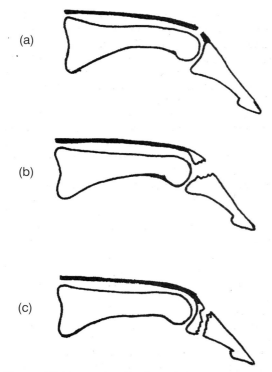

Figure 4.5. Types of mallet finger injury: (a) rupture of distal extensor tendon; (b) avulsion fracture of the base of the distal phalanx; (c) fracture separation of epiphysis of distal phalanx.

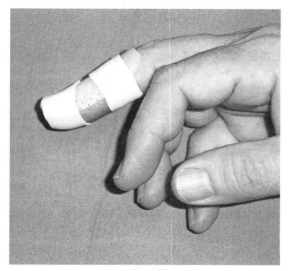

Figure 4.6. A closed mallet finger injury is treated with 6 weeks of immobilization. The DIP joint is maintained in full extension with a thermoplastic splint that can be worn volarly or dorsally. The splint should allow full PIP joint flexion range.

A layer of paper tape (e.g. Micropore or Hypafix) applied to the skin prior to splint application will help prevent maceration. If the distal joint is swollen, as is often the case with an associated avulsion fracture, the splint may need to be adjusted until swelling has stabilized. Coban used beneath the splint will hasten resolution of oedema. Full PIP joint mobility should be maintained throughout this period.

If the patient demonstrates joint hypermobility, the splint can hold the DIP joint in slight hyperextension where this position can be gained with ease. Hypermobile joints often require prolonged splinting, i.e. an additional 3 to 4 weeks. Whether the joint is splinted in neutral extension or slight hyperextension, care is taken to avoid restricting the circulation. The patient is instructed in skin and splint care. The splint should be removed at least once each day to 'air' the finger and to check for adverse effects from the splint. The patient must ensure that the DIP joint is supported in full extension whenever the splint is removed. While the splint is off, the skin is gently tapped and massaged to stimulate the circulation.

Following the immobilization period, gentle active DIP joint flexion exercises are commenced. Night and intermittent day splinting is maintained for a further 2 weeks. The patient attempts gentle unforced composite IP joint flexion. The finger is then straightened from the flexed position and extension range of the distal joint is carefully assessed for any sign of lag. Exercise sessions are performed every 2 h with 5 to 10 repetitions. A desirable DIP joint flexion range during the first week is 20 to 30 degrees. The goal is then to achieve a further 10 degrees during each ensuing week. Patients who demonstrate significant flexion range when the splint is removed tend to be more prone to a recurrence of the deformity. If the DIP joint flexion deformity appears to be recurring, extension splinting is reinstituted for a further 2 weeks when the situation is reassessed. Resisted activities are avoided until the 10th week.

If the mallet deformity has resulted in a secondary swan-neck deformity (i.e. the PIP joint has assumed a posture of hyperextension in association with the flexion deformity at the DIP joint), then both IP joints will need to be included in the splint. The PIP joint is placed in 35 to 45 degrees of flexion to advance the lateral bands, while the DIP joint is held in neutral extension.

Open injury

Open wounds are best treated by repair and internal fixation of the distal joint with a K-wire which is removed 2 to 3 weeks later. An extension splint is then applied for a further 3 to 4 weeks. Oedema in the distal segment of the finger is managed with Coban wrap (25 mm). Management is then as for closed mallet injury.

Zones III and IV

Conservative management for closed injury

Injury to the extensor tendon mechanism over the PIP joint can produce a buttonhole deformity which, if untreated, becomes a fixed deformity with PIP joint flexion contracture and DIP joint hyperextension contracture (Fig. 4.7).

This deformity results when the lateral bands fall below the axis of the PIP joint. When this occurs, the lateral bands become flexors of the joint while at the same time concentrating their extension force at the DIP joint. Shortening of the oblique retinacular ligaments quickly ensues. This further compounds loss of DIP flexion range which is often the most disabling aspect of this deformity.

Suspected closed injuries of the central slip are treated by splinting which maintains the PIP joint in full extension for a period of 6 weeks. The DIP joint is left free to move. A variety of splints can be used to achieve this goal, e.g. thermoplastic finger splint, Capener or a circumferential plaster cast. Because the finger is frequently swollen, a plaster cast is the splint of choice (Fig. 4.8). This will provide gentle even compression and will alleviate joint discomfort. The cast may need to be changed every few days until swelling has fully settled. The cast should not impede DIP joint flexion which should be carried out passively and actively on an hourly basis with 10 to 20 repetitions. In most cases, it can be left in place for about 10 days before it softens and needs replacing.

If the deformity presents late, serial casting is used to overcome the flexion deformity prior to the 6-week splinting period which will begin when neutral extension range has been achieved. Gentle dynamic flexion splinting of the DIP joint can be incorporated into the plaster to overcome tightness of the oblique retinacular ligament.

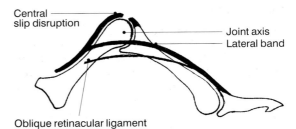

Figure 4.7. Buttonhole deformity following injury to the central slip of the extensor tendon. The lateral bands fall below the axis of the PIP joint and become flexors of this joint. Their extension force at the DIP joint becomes more concentrated, resulting in DIP joint hyperextension.

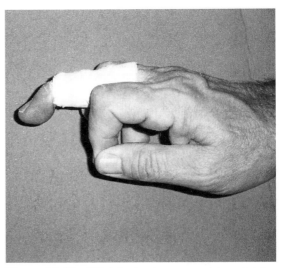

Figure 4.8. The PIP joint is plaster-casted to maintain full extension. In the presence of a flexion contracture, serial casting is undertaken until full extension range has been regained. The 6-week splinting period is then commenced from that time. Passive and active DIP joint exercises are performed hourly.

Gentle unresisted active PIP joint flexion/extension exercises are commenced after 6 weeks of extension splinting. Night splinting in a thermoplastic finger splint is maintained for a further 2 weeks. Flexion of the PIP joint should be regained gradually over a number of weeks. Forced flexion of the joint will result in attenuation of the tendon and a recurrence of the deformity.

Open injury

The traditional postoperative treatment following repair in Zones III and IV has involved immobilization of the PIP joint for a 6-week period. Due to the significant tendon-bone interface and proximity to joint structures, this area is particularly prone to adhesion formation resulting in restricted tendon excursion, extensor lag and joint stiffness (Newport et al., 1990). Implementation of the active short arc motion protocol as proposed by Evans (1994) has shown statistically superior results when compared with traditional management of these zones.

The author has now used this protocol for several years with good results. Minor modifications to the original protocol have been made. These include:

1. A dorsal finger splint rather than a volar one.
2. The use of only one template (instead of two) during active exercise; the author does not use the second template used for active DIP joint flexion exercises.

Active short arc motion protocol

Within a day or two of surgery, the interphalangeal joints are fitted with a thermoplastic finger splint that maintains both joints in full extension (i.e. 0 degrees). Maintenance of the fully extended position between exercise sessions is most important in avoiding elongation of the tendon (Fig. 4.9).

To help eliminate digital oedema, the finger is wrapped in a single layer of Coban (25 mm)

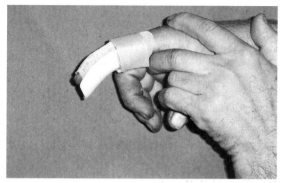

Figure 4.10. The volar template splint allows 30 and 25 degrees of active flexion at the PIP and DIP joints, respectively. The wrist should be maintained in 30 degrees of flexion and the MCP joints maintained in neutral extension during the manoeuvre.

applied over a non-bulky dressing in a distal to proximal direction. The initial splint may need to be replaced if postoperative swelling has been significant.

A volar template splint is then made which will accommodate 30 degrees of active PIP joint flexion and 25 degrees of active DIP joint flexion (Fig. 4.10). This splint is used every waking hour. The prescribed exercises are performed with the wrist in 30 degrees of flexion and the MCP joint in neutral extension or slight flexion. With the volar template splint held in place, the patient flexes both IP joints to the limit of the splint and then actively extends the digit to neutral extension at both IP joints. The position of extension is held for

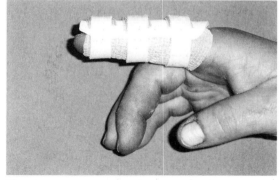

Figure 4.9. One or two days following open repair of the extensor tendon in Zone III or IV, the digit is fitted with a thermoplastic finger splint that maintains both IP joints in full extension. Coban wrap is used over the dressing to treat postoperative oedema.

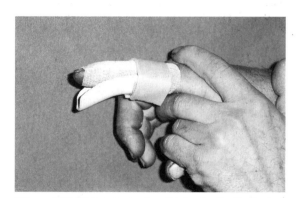

Figure 4.11. Following active flexion to the limit of the volar splint, both IP joints are then actively extended to neutral extension. This extended position is held for several seconds before the manoeuvre is repeated.

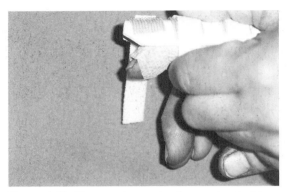

Figure 4.12. The exercise session is completed with active stabilized DIP joint flexion/extension exercises which maintain DIP joint mobility and excursion of the lateral bands and oblique retinacular ligament. If the lateral bands have been repaired, active DIP joint flexion is limited to 30 degrees for the first two weeks. The PIP joint must be kept in full extension during DIP joint exercises.

several seconds prior to again flexing to the limit of the splint (Fig. 4.11). This manoeuvre is repeated 20 times every hour.

The other component of the hourly exercise routine involves active flexion of the DIP joint with the PIP joint held in full extension. This can be performed by undoing the distal strap of the splint and stabilizing the PIP joint during active flexion of the distal joint (Fig. 4.12). Movement of this joint is important in maintaining excursion of the lateral bands and the oblique retinacular ligaments. If the lateral bands have not been repaired, the distal joint is fully flexed and extended. Where they have undergone repair, active DIP joint flexion is limited to 30 degrees and is followed by active DIP joint extension. This exercise is repeated 10 to 15 times.

If no extensor lag has developed, the volar template splint is modified or replaced after 2 weeks to allow 40 degrees of PIP joint flexion during the described manoeuvre. This is increased to 50 degrees by week 3, and to 70 or 80 degrees by the end of the 4th week.

Static extension splinting between hourly exercise sessions is maintained for 6 weeks. Composite active finger flexion can begin at the end of the 5th week. Return of flexion range should be gradual so as not to jeopardize PIP joint extension range. Fully resisted activity is avoided until the 10th week.

Zones V and VI

These two zones lie between the MCP joints and the extensor retinaculum. Closed injuries to the sagittal hood system over the MCP joints can occur with blunt trauma and result in an extensor lag or ulnar drift of the tendon. These injuries are treated by splinting the involved MCP joint in neutral extension for a period of 4 to 6 weeks.

Tendon glide is more readily restored in these proximal zones because this area has greater soft tissue mobility. Nonetheless, adhesion of the repaired tendon to skin and bone does still occur, particularly if the injury has involved other structures, e.g. bone and intrinsic musculature, following a crush injury.

Because the dorsum of the hand can accommodate significant swelling, the propensity toward adhesion formation is great. Prompt management of postoperative oedema is important in minimizing the risk of these adhesions.

Postoperative management

As for Zones III and IV, tendon injuries in these zones can be managed by:

1. Static splinting and immobilization.
2. Dynamic splinting and early controlled motion.

The controlled motion protocol in these zones was originally devised by Evans to overcome problems associated with complex injuries. Because of the undisputed biochemical and biomechanical advantages associated with early controlled motion, Evans now also uses the dynamic approach with the simple tendon injury. Since starting on the dynamic protocol four years ago, this author has not used the static splinting method other than for patients considered unable to cope with the regimen. Both methods of management will be described.

1. Static splint and immobilization

On the 2nd or 3rd postoperative day the plaster is replaced with a volar thermoplastic splint which maintains the wrist in 45 degrees of extension and the MCP joints in 0 to 20 degrees of flexion. The interphalangeal joints are maintained in full extension with a distal splint component that is removed for IP joint exercises. The maintenance of IP joint extension is important in preventing palmar plate

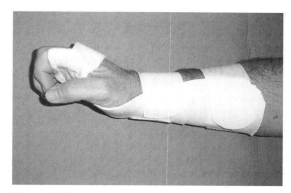

Figure 4.13. Postoperative splint following extensor tendon repair for Zones V and VI using the static immobilization protocol. A removable distal component (not shown) is worn at night and between exercise sessions to prevent flexion deformity at the interphalangeal joints. Full active IP joint flexion should be possible within the splint.

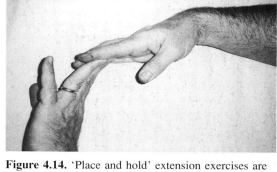

Figure 4.14. 'Place and hold' extension exercises are performed with the wrist in 20 to 30 degrees of flexion while the fingers are supported in full extension. The supporting hand is then removed and the patient is asked to maintain active digital extension for several seconds.

contracture and subsequent flexion deformity. The splint extends from two-thirds along the forearm to just proximal to the PIP joints so IP joint flexion can be performed (Fig. 4.13).

Days 3 to 24

Because IP joint motion produces only minimal extensor tendon excursion in Zones V and VI (Brand and Hollister, 1993), active IP joint flexion exercises are performed every 2 h with 10 repetitions. These are followed by IP joint passive extension. The distal component of the splint is worn between exercise sessions to maintain full digital extension.

When the sutures are removed after about 10 days, the hand is bathed in warm, soapy water (with care taken to maintain the correct position of wrist and finger extension) and gentle oil massage is begun. Scar is managed with silicone gel which is worn beneath Tubigrip elastic stocking. All traces of oil are removed prior to application of the gel.

Day 24 onwards

At $3\frac{1}{2}$ weeks, gentle active motion of the MCP joints is commenced. The following exercises are performed:

1. Because wrist flexion is synergistic with finger extension, active MCP joint extension exercises are performed with the wrist in 20 to 30 degrees

of flexion. This position reduces the passive tension of the opposing extrinsic digital flexors. 'Place and hold' exercises are performed with the wrist supported in 20 to 30 degrees of flexion and the fingers supported in full extension (Fig. 4.14). The supporting hand is then removed from the fingers and the patient is asked to maintain active digital extension with minimal exertion for several seconds before relaxing. The patient is then asked to actively flex the MCP joints to 30 degrees, hold this position for several seconds, and then actively extend the MCP joints to neutral extension. This exercise is repeated 10 to 20 times every 1 to 2 hours.

2. The wrist is then extended to 45 degrees and the patient attempts 40 to 60 degrees of MCP joint flexion with the IP joints maintained in extension, i.e. the 'intrinsic-plus' position.

3. The third exercise involves active flexion and extension of the IP joints with the wrist in 20 to 30 degrees of extension and MCP joints held in neutral extension range.

At week 4, composite flexion (i.e. all three finger joints flexing simultaneously), is begun with the wrist held in 45 degrees of extension. Protective splinting is maintained between exercise sessions until the end of the 6th week.

At week 6, extrinsic extension exercises are added to the programme. This involves extending the MCP joints while maintaining maximum IP joint flexion and is performed with the wrist in neutral extension. The patient can engage in light unresisted daily activity at this stage.

If MCP joint flexion range is still restricted by the 8th week, a gentle dynamic MCP joint flexion splint is applied. Fully resisted activity is avoided until week 12 when the repair will have sufficient tensile strength.

2. Dynamic splinting and early controlled motion

A dorsal forearm-based dynamic extension splint is fitted to the patient within the first 3 days of surgery. This splint holds the wrist in 40 to 45 degrees of extension. Dynamic traction (using rubber bands that are connected to nylon thread), maintain the MCP and IP joints at 0 degrees (or neutral) extension range. The tension of the rubber bands is checked daily to ensure that neutral extension range is being maintained (Fig. 4.15).

To help maintain IP joint extension at rest and during active MCP joint flexion exercises, the finger slings will need to be fairly wide and extend distal to the PIP joints. Narrow slings that sit beneath the proximal phalanx only, will allow the IP joints to assume a flexed position. When the patient then attempts active MCP joint flexion exercises, there will be a strong tendency for flexion to occur at the already flexed IP joints, rather than at the MCP joints. In other words, the patient will be practising extrinsic IP joint flexion exercises rather than intrinsic MCP joint flexion exercises. If wide finger slings do not prevent the IP joints from assuming a flexed posture, thin thermoplastic finger splints used inside the finger

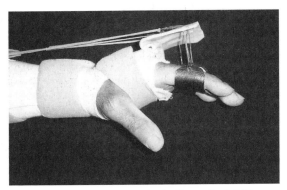

Figure 4.16. The patient actively flexes the MCP joints to a limit of 30 degrees every hour. The joints are returned to neutral extension by the rubber band traction. This manoeuvre is repeated 20 times at each hourly exercise session.

slings and held on with Microfoam tape will overcome this problem. Alternatively, small wooden 'paddle-pop' sticks can be inserted under the digit during MCP joint exercise sessions.

On an hourly basis, the patient actively flexes the MCP joints to a limit of 30 degrees and then allows the rubber band traction to return the MCP joints to neutral extension (Fig. 4.16). This manoeuvre is repeated 20 times. The author of this protocol (Evans, 1989) uses a volar blocking component during exercise to limit active flexion to 30 degrees. Our patients are provided with a line diagram depicting the desired angle. Prior to commencing the exercise, the manoeuvre is practised on the opposite hand until the patient understands what is required. As a departure from the original protocol which has the MCP joints flexing to a limit of 30 degrees for the first 3 weeks, our patients are asked to flex to 45 degrees after 2 weeks and to 60 degrees after 4 weeks. Splinting is maintained for a total of 6 weeks.

Maintenance of interphalangeal joint flexibility is important throughout the splinting period. Gentle active IP joint flexion exercises can be carried out with the wrist and MCP joints maintained in extension. Flexion of the IP joints in this position creates only minimal excursion of the extensor tendon in Zones V and VI. Gentle active IP joint flexion exercises are performed 4 to 6 times daily with 5 to 10 repetitions.

The finger slings are removed for this exercise and the MCP joints are maintained in full extension. This can be effectively accomplished by holding a pen across the base of the proximal phalanges. This

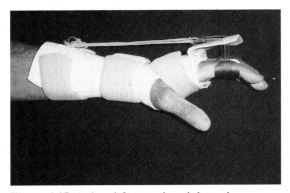

Figure 4.15. A dorsal forearm-based dynamic extension splint is fitted on the 3rd postoperative day. The digital slings maintain the MCP joints in neutral extension range.

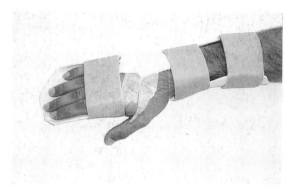

Figure 4.17. A static volar splint can be used at night if the patient finds the dynamic splint awkward to sleep in.

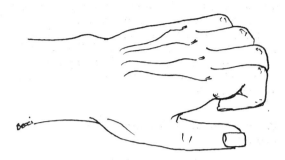

Figure 4.18. Extrinsic EDC extension exercises are performed by extending the MCP joints from the fisted position, i.e. interphalangeal joint flexion is maintained while the patient actively extends the MCP joints.

will accommodate almost complete IP joint flexion range while allowing good visualization of the MCP joints to ensure that they are maintained in full extension. The IP joints are then passively extended after each flexion exercise.

At night, the patient uses either a static volar splint that maintains the wrist and fingers in extension or a volar finger segment is added to the dynamic splint so that digital extension is maintained (Fig. 4.17).

The majority of patients are able to demonstrate full composite flexion following removal of the splint at 6 weeks and extensor lag is rarely seen. Where lag is present, extrinsic extension exercises are instituted. Patients should avoid fully resisted activity until 12 weeks following repair (Fig. 4.18).

Minimal active muscle-tendon tension (Evans and Thompson, 1993)

This manoeuvre is the corollary of the 'place and hold' exercise used in the early active motion protocol following flexor tendon repair. It is based on the tenodesis effect resulting from the synergistic action between the wrist extensors and the finger flexors (Savage, 1988). The converse situation, i.e. that wrist flexion is synergistic with finger extension, is utilized following extensor tendon injury.

If minimal active muscle-tendon tension (MAMTT) is to be incorporated into the therapy programme, it should be done so within 24 h of surgery before collagen bonds, which would limit tendon glide, have formed (Gelberman et al., 1985).

It has been experimentally demonstrated that the expected reduction in tensile strength following repair can possibly be prevented if the repair site undergoes very early stress (Amiel et al., 1991).

Just as full passive IP joint flexion should be achieved prior to the commencement of active flexion following flexor tendon repair, so too, full passive extension of all three digital joints is a prerequisite to the commencement of 'place and hold' active extension exercises. Full passive mobility into extension reduces the resistance of the antagonistic flexors. Resistance is also created by dorsal hand oedema. For this reason, a gentle compression bandage should be used postoperatively to help control and eliminate oedema promptly.

MAMTT is practised only in therapy. The therapist supports the patient's wrist in 20 degrees of flexion and all digital joints in 0 degrees extension. Our patients are exercised into slight hyperextension if the opposite hand exhibits any degree of hypermobility. When the finger joints can be placed in neutral extension with ease (i.e. no resistance is perceived during passive extension), the therapist removes the supporting hand from the digits and asks the patient to maintain the extended position with minimal active effort for several seconds. The fingers are then relaxed and the MCP joints fall into a position of about 30 degrees of flexion. The patient is then asked to actively extend the MCP joints to neutral (0 degrees) extension and again, maintain the extended position for several seconds. This manoeuvre is repeated 20 times before the hand is returned to the splint.

Zone VII

At this level the extensor tendons pass beneath the extensor retinaculum. Here the tendons are prone to proximal retraction. Repaired tendons in this area have a tendency to adhere to one another as well as to the adjacent extensor retinaculum. Scarring is usually significant in this zone following repair. Silicone gel is applied to scar as soon as the wound has healed.

If wrist extensors alone have been repaired (i.e. ECRL, ECRB or ECU), the wrist is splinted into 40 to 45 degrees of extension for a period of 5 weeks while the fingers are left free to move. Active wrist flexion exercises are commenced after this time.

If finger or thumb extensors are involved, the aftercare is the same as for Zones V and VI in the digits, and III, IV and V for thumb zones (see below).

Injury to the thumb extensors

Zone I

Zone I is the area over the IP joint. Mallet thumb is quite rare. Closed injuries are treated with continuous IP joint extension (or slight hyperextension where possible) splinting for 8 weeks. Tendon laceration in this zone is repaired and followed by 6 weeks of extension splinting. A further 2 weeks of intermittent splinting is maintained after IP joint flexion exercises have been commenced. See 'Zones I and II' (fingers) for exercise protocol.

Zone II

This zone involves the proximal phalanx and injury to the tendon is usually secondary to laceration or a crush injury rather than avulsion. Because the tendon has increased width in this zone and curves over the phalanx, it usually sustains only partial laceration. If the laceration involves less than 50 per cent of the tendon, the injury is treated conservatively with a dressing and support splinting of the IP joint. Gentle active motion is commenced after 10 days. Support splinting between exercises is maintained for 4 to 6 weeks.

Surgical repair is carried out for more significant lacerations. The thumb IP joint is then splinted in full extension for 6 weeks. See 'Zones I and II' (fingers) for exercise protocol.

Zones III, IV and V

Zone III is the area over the MCP joint and may involve one or both of the thumb extensors (i.e. EPL or EPB). The tendons in this area are sufficiently thick to allow the use of standard core-type sutures.

Zone IV is the area over the metacarpal. Zone V is in the region of the extensor retinaculum and injury to the EPL in this zone is considered complex because the tendon is synovial at this level. Evans (1995) advocates that management of the tendon in this zone should involve early controlled passive motion and/or MAMTT exercises because dense adhesions at this level often limit excursion of the repaired tendon.

1. Static splinting and immobilization

If the immobilization method is used postoperatively, a static splint is fitted which holds the wrist in 40 degrees of extension and the thumb in radial abduction with the MCP and IP thumb joints in neutral extension (Fig. 4.19). If only the EPB tendon is involved, the IP joint is left free to move. A distal component, holding the IP joint in extension at night, is added to the splint to avoid the IP joint developing a flexion deformity. Care should be taken to avoid placing the MCP joint in hyperextension. The fingers are left free to move.

Between the 3rd and 4th week, the splint is removed every 2 h for gentle active thumb exercises. Gentle active thumb joint flexion is

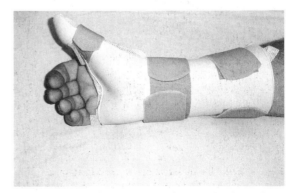

Figure 4.19. The static postoperative splint for EPL repair holds the wrist in 40 degrees of extension and the thumb in radial abduction. The thumb MCP and IP joints are held in neutral extension. In the case of hypermobile patients, care should be taken to avoid hyperextension of the MCP joint during splint fitting.

practised with the wrist held in maximum extension. Active thumb extension is not performed with the wrist held in extension. 'Place and hold' MAMTT thumb extension exercises are commenced by allowing the wrist to go into 15 to 20 degrees of flexion while holding the thumb in full extension, see p. 53. The support is then withdrawn from the thumb and the patient gently holds the extended thumb position with minimal effort for several seconds. These exercises are repeated 5 to 10 times during the first week after which repetitions are increased.

When the splint is removed after 6 weeks, the thumb can be actively exercised with the wrist in all positions. Due to periarticular thickening, regaining flexion at the MCP joint can sometimes be difficult. If this is the case, gentle dynamic flexion splinting can be instituted between the 6th and 7th week.

2. Dynamic splinting with controlled mobilization: used for Zones III, IV and V following EPL repair

The dynamic splint maintains the wrist and thumb in the following position:

1. Wrist in 40 degrees of extension.
2. CMC joint in neutral extension.
3. MCP joint in 0 degrees extension.
4. IP joint at 0 degrees extension.

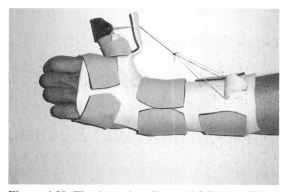

Figure 4.20. The dynamic splint used following EPL repair in Zones III, IV and V holds the thumb IP joint is held in a position of neutral extension by rubber band traction. The patient actively flexes the IP joint to 60 degrees every hour with 20 repetitions. After each active flexion exercise, the patient relaxes the thumb and allows the rubber band traction to return the joint to neutral extension.

The dynamic traction sling is applied to the distal phalanx (Fig. 4.20). The patient performs active IP joint flexion to a range of 60 degrees every hour during the day. This results in 5 mm of tendon excursion at Lister's tubercle. The rubber band traction returns the IP joint to neutral extension. If the patient finds the dynamic splint awkward during sleep, a static splint is used at night. Care is taken to avoid a posture of hyperextension at the MCP joint.

The 'place and hold' MAMTT exercises described in the previous section can be employed after the first day of surgery with the permission of the treating surgeon.

After the 3rd week, gentle active MCP joint flexion is commenced out of the splint with the wrist maintained in extension. By the 5th week, composite thumb flexion and opposition with the wrist in extension can be begun. After the 6th week, movements of the thumb can be practised with the wrist in all positions. Protective splinting between exercise sessions is maintained for 6 weeks. The thumb should not be involved in fully resisted activity until after the 12th week.

References

Amiel, D., Gelberman, R., Harwood, F. and Siegel, D. (1991). Fibronectin in healing flexor tendons subjected to immobilization or early controlled passive motion. *Matrix II.*, **11**, 184–9.

Boyes, J. H. (1970). *Bunnell's Surgery of the Hand.* J. B. Lippincott.

Brand, P. W. and Hollister, A. (1993). *Clinical Mechanics of the Hand.* Mosby Year Book.

Browne, E. Z. and Ribik, C. A. (1989). Early dynamic splinting for extensor tendon injuries. *J. Hand Surg.*, **14A**, 72.

Duran, R. J. and Houser, R. G. (1975). Controlled passive motion following flexor tendon repair in zones II and III. In *The American Academy of Orthopaedic Surgeons: Symposium on tendon surgery in the hand.* Mosby.

Elliot, D. and McGrouther, D. A. (1986). The excursions of the long extensor tendons of the hand. *J. Hand Surg.*, **11B**, 77–80.

Evans, R. B. (1994). Early active short arc motion for the repaired central slip. *J. Hand Surg.*, **19A**, 991–7.

Evans, R. B. (1995). An update on extensor tendon management. In *Rehabilitation of the Hand: Surgery and Therapy* (J. M. Hunter, E. J. Mackin and A. D. Callahan, eds) pp. 565–606, Mosby.

Evans, R. B. and Burkhalter, W. E. (1986). A study of the dynamic anatomy of extensor tendons and implications for treatment. *J. Hand Surg.*, **11A**, 774–9.

Evans, R. B. and Thompson, D. E. (1993). The application of stress to the healing tendon. *J. Hand Ther.*, **6**, 262–80.

Gelberman, R. H., Vande Berg, J. S., Manske, P. R. and Akeson, W. H. (1985). The early stages of flexor tendon healing: A morphologic study of the first fourteen days. *J. Hand Surg.,* **10A**, 776–84.

Gelberman, R. H., Botte, M., Spiegelman, J. and Akeson, W. (1986). The excursion and deformation of repaired flexor tendons treated with protected early motion. *J. Hand Surg.,* **11A**, 106–10.

Harris, C. Jr. and Rutledge, G. L. Jr. (1972). The functional anatomy of the extensor mechanism of the finger. *J. Bone Joint Surg.,* **54A**, 713.

Hung, L. K., Chan, A., Chang, J. et al., (1990). Early controlled active mobilization with dynamic splintage for treatment of extensor tendon injuries. *J. Hand Surg.,* **15A**, 251–7.

Kleinert, H. E. and Verdan, C. (1983). Report of the committee on tendon injuries. *J. Hand Surg.,* **8A**, 794–8.

Newport, M. L., Blair, W. F. and Steyers, C. M. Jr. (1990). Long-term results of extensor tendon repair. *J. Hand Surg.,* **15A**, 961–6.

Newport, M. L., Pollack, G. R. and Williams, C. D. (1995). Biomechanical characteristics of suture techniques in extensor Zone IV. *J. Hand Surg.,* **20A**, 650–6.

Saldana, M. J., Choban, S., Westerbeck, P. and Schacherer, T. G. (1991). Results of acute Zone III extensor tendon injuries treated with dynamic extension splinting. *J. Hand Surg.,* **16A**, 1145–50.

Savage, R. (1988). The influence of wrist position on the minimum force required for active movement of the interphalangeal joints. *J. Hand Surg.,* **13B**, 262–8.

Further reading

Bendz, P. (1985). The functional significance of the oblique retinacular ligament of Landsmeer. A review and new proposals. *J. Hand Surg.,* **10B**, 25.

Chow, J. A., Dovelle, S, Thomas, L. J. and Callahan, D. (1987). Postoperative management of repair of extensor tendons of the hand-dynamic splinting versus static splinting. *Orthop. Trans.,* **11**, 258–9.

Chow, J. A., Dovelle, S., Thomas, L. J., Ho, P. K. and Saldana, J. (1989). A comparison of results of extensor tendon repair followed by early controlled mobilization versus static immobilization. *J. Hand Surg.,* **14B**, 18–20.

Doyle, J. R. (1999). Extensor tendons-acute injuries. In *Green's Operative Hand Surgery* (D. P. Green, R. N. Hotchkiss and W. C. Pederson, eds) pp. 1950–87, Mosby.

Eaton, R. G. (1969). The extensor mechanism of the fingers. *Bull. Hosp. Joint Dis.,* **30**, 39–47.

Elson, R. A. (1986). Rupture of the central slip of the extensor hood of the finger: a test for early diagnosis. *J. Bone Joint Surg.,* **68B**, 229.

Evans, R. B. (1986). Therapeutic management of extensor tendon injuries. *Hand Clin.,* **2**, 157–69.

Evans, R. B. (1989). Clinical application of controlled stress to the healing extensor tendon: a review of 122 cases. *Phys. Ther.,* **68(12)**, 1041–9.

Evans, R. B. and Thompson, D. E. (1992). An analysis of factors that support early active short arc motion of the repaired central slip. *J. Hand Ther.,* **5**, 187–201.

Ishizuki, M. (1990). Traumatic and spontaneous dislocation of extensor tendon of the long finger. *J. Hand Surg.,* **15A**, 967–72.

Kim, P. T., Aoki, M., Tokita, F. and Ishii, S. (1996). Tensile strength of cross-stitch epitenon suture. *J. Hand Surg.,* **21B**, 821–3.

Landsmeer, J. M. F. (1949). Anatomy of the dorsal aponeurosis of the human finger and its functional significance. *Anat. Rec.,* **104**, 31–44.

Littler, J. W. (1967). The finger extensor mechanism. *Surg. Clin. North Am.,* **47**, 415.

Maddy, L. S. and Meyerdierks, E. M. (1997). Dynamic extension assist splinting of acute central slip lacerations. *J. Hand Ther.,* **10**, 206–12.

Masson, J. A. (1999). Hand IV: extensor tendons, rheumatoid arthritis and Dupuytren's disease. *Selected Readings in Plast. Surg.,* **8(35)**, 1–20.

Miura, T., Nakamura, R. and Torii, S. (1986). Conservative treatment for a ruptured extensor tendon on the dorsum of the proximal phalanges of the thumb (mallet thumb). *J. Hand Surg.,* **11A**, 229–33.

Newport, M. L. and Shukla, A. (1992). Electrophysiologic basis of dynamic extensor splinting. *J. Hand Surg.,* **17A**, 272.

Patel, M. R., Lipson, L. B. and Desai, S. S. (1986). Conservative treatment of mallet thumb. *J. Hand Surg.,* **11A**, 45–7.

Rayan, G. M. and Mullins, P. T. (1987). Skin necrosis complicating mallet finger splinting and vascularity of the distal interphalangeal joint overlying skin. *J. Hand Surg.,* **12A**, 548–52.

Stern, P. J. and Kastrup, J. J. (1988). Complications and prognosis of treatment of mallet finger. *J. Hand Surg.,* **13A**, 32.

von Schroeder, H. P. and Botte, M. J. (1993). The functional significance of the long extensors and juncturae tendinum in finger extension. *J. Hand Surg.,* **18A**, 641–7.

von Schroeder, H. P. and Botte, M. J. (1995). Anatomy of the extensor tendons of the fingers: variations and multiplicity. *J. Hand Surg.,* **20A**, 27–34.

5

Peripheral nerve injuries

Anatomy and pathophysiology

Peripheral nerves are complex composite structures comprised of nerve fibres, connective tissue and blood vessels. The nerve fibres (or axons) extend from the nerve cell body to the receptor organs in the motor and sensory endplates (Fig. 5.1). The peripheral nerve carries three types of nerve fibres, i.e. motor, sensory and autonomic. The proportion of fibres in each nerve depends on the function of that nerve. In the upper limb, the median nerve has the greatest proportion of autonomic fibres. Motor nerve fibres originate from cell bodies in the ventral horn of the spinal cord and terminate at the neuromuscular junction. Sensory fibres originate from cell bodies in the dorsal root ganglia and terminate at receptors such as Pacinian corpuscles, Meissner's corpuscles or as free nerve endings.

Various substances, e.g. proteins, enzymes, free amino acids, polypeptides, etc., are synthesized within the cell body and are necessary for the normal function and survival of the axon. Axoplasmic transport mechanisms move these substances to the periphery (antegrade transport) where breakdown products are then returned in a proximal direction (retrograde transport). The axonal transport occurs at speeds that vary from about 1–400 mm per day (Weiss and Gorio, 1982).

Most peripheral nerve axons are covered by a myelin sheath which is produced by flattened cells known as Schwann cells. Unmyelinated fibres are mainly small sensory fibres that conduct pain impulses from the skin. The unmyelinated gaps between the segments of the myelin sheath are called nodes of Ranvier and are about 1–2 mm apart. This discontinuity in the myelin sheath allows rapid impulse conduction as the action potential leaps from one node to the next (Fig. 5.2).

Endoneurium

There are successive layers of connective tissue surrounding the nerve fibres. The endoneurium is the supporting collagenous tissue of the individual fibres. It takes part in the formation of the 'endoneurial tube' which contains the myelinated axon and associated Schwann cells.

Perineurium

The nerve fibres with their related endoneurium form aggregations called bundles, fasciculi or funiculi which are the smallest units of the nerve that can be surgically manipulated. Fascicles are enclosed by the next connective tissue layer, the perineurium. This thin, lamellated sheath protects the contents of the endoneurial tubes, acts as a mechanical barrier to external forces and provides a diffusion barrier that keeps certain substances out of the intrafascicular environment (Lundborg, 1988). This sheath has great mechanical strength and strongly resists longitudinal traction.

Epineurium

The epineurium is the outermost layer and is located between the fascicles and superficially in the nerve. The epineurium cushions the fascicles from external pressure and allows movement of

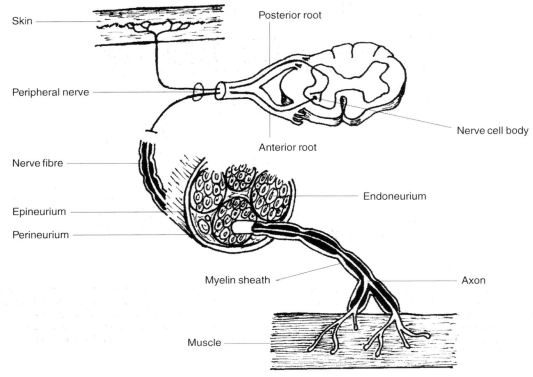

Figure 5.1. Anatomy of a nerve cell showing the cell body and the nerve fibre (axon) with its component parts. (From Grabb, 1970, with permission.)

one fascicle upon another. The amount of epineurial connective tissue can vary enormously (25–75%) among nerves and at different levels within the same nerve (Sunderland and Bradley, 1949). The epineurium is often more abundant in areas requiring greater protection such as where the nerve is in close proximity to bone or a joint (Sunderland, 1978).

Nerve vasculature

The peripheral nerve contains vascular networks in the epineurium, the perineurium and the endoneurium. The blood supply to the peripheral nerve as a whole is provided by large vessels that approach the nerve segmentally along its course. Upon reaching the nerve, these vessels divide into ascending and

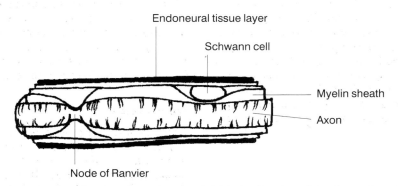

Figure 5.2. Most peripheral nerves are covered by a myelin sheath. The unmyelinated gaps between the segments of the myelin sheath are called nodes of Ranvier.

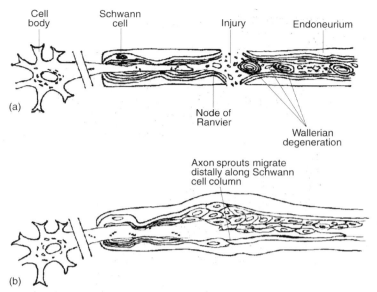

Figure 5.3. (a) Nerve degeneration. When there has been axonal disruption, there is degeneration of the axon and myelin sheath distal to the wound and proximally, as far as the next node of Ranvier. Degeneration is initiated by the ingrowth of macrophages which, together with the Schwann cells, clear the endoneurial tube of debris in preparation for axon regeneration. (b) Nerve regeneration. The cell body and proximal axon stump enlarge to satisfy the metabolic requirements for regeneration. The budding axons grow toward the distal segment and advance along the Schwann cell columns.

descending branches that run longitudinally and frequently anastomose with the vessels in the perineurium and epineurium. The microvascular system has a large reserve capacity because axonal transport and impulse propagation depend on a local oxygen supply (Lundborg, 1975).

Types of nerve injury

Nerves can be injured through trauma (laceration, crush or burn), compression (acute or chronic), stretching (traction), ischaemia, electrical current or the late effects of radiation. The more common nerve injuries are those involving lacerations which can be either partial or complete.

Sir Herbert Seddon has described three levels of injury: neurapraxia, axonotmesis and neurotmesis. The classification described by Sir Sidney Sunderland has five categories of injury, the 1st, 2nd and 5th of which correspond to the above three, respectively.

Neurapraxia

Neurapraxia is the mildest form of nerve injury and axonal continuity is maintained. This injury involves a localized block to conduction; however, proximally and distally to the lesion, nerve conduction is preserved. A full recovery is expected and is usually complete within weeks or several months.

Axonotmesis

Axonotmesis is a more severe form of nerve injury with disruption to the continuity of axons within the nerve. Because there has been axonal disruption, Wallerian degeneration of the distal axon will occur. There should, however, be good functional recovery because the supportive connective tissue remains intact so that axonal regeneration is specific to the end organ. Functional recovery can take some months depending on the level of the disruption and how far regeneration needs to occur.

Neurotmesis

Seddon's last category of nerve injury, i.e. neurotmesis, refers to a complete transection of the nerve with loss of integrity of the perineurium and epineurium and corresponds to the 5th category described by Sunderland. The 3rd and 4th levels of injury in the Sunderland classification refer to varying degrees of intraneural disruption and loss of fascicular integrity that can result from moderate to severe traction and crushing injuries where the epineurium remains intact. Even if the perineurium has remained intact, intraneural haemorrhaging and oedema will often result in scar tissue formation, making nerve regeneration less likely.

Degeneration and regeneration

1. Wallerian degeneration

Degeneration of the distal axon begins at the level of injury. The interruption to the flow of axoplasm results in an accumulation of axoplasmic substances at the proximal stump, where degeneration occurs only as far as the next node of Ranvier. Degeneration is initiated by the ingrowth of macrophages which trigger the proliferation of Schwann cells. The macrophages and Schwann cells clear the Schwann cell tube of myelin and axoplasm in readiness for subsequent axon regeneration (Stoll et al., 1989) (Fig. 5.3(a)).

2. Axon regeneration

Severed axons begin to send out a great number of sprouts within six hours of injury. This occurs proximal to the nerve lesion, at the most distal remaining node of Ranvier. These initial sprouts are usually resorbed; however, permanent sprouts are formed a day later. These grow towards the distal segment and then advance along the endoneurial tubes (or Schwann cell columns). The regulation of axon growth and orientation is complex and reliant on a variety of biochemical and biomechanical mechanisms. The maximum rate of axonal outgrowth in humans is about 1 mm per day (Fig. 5.3(b)).

Effect on associated tissues

Muscle changes

Muscle fibres usually undergo moderate to severe atrophy by three months and moderate to severe fibrosis after about one year. The degree of atrophy and fibrosis varies significantly among individuals and can be affected by infection, muscle stretching, muscle nutrition or the age of the patient. After a three-year period, muscle fibres exhibit progressive fragmentation and disintegration, with the muscle fibres gradually being replaced by fibrotic tissue (Bowden and Gutmann, 1944).

Sensory loss

A completely severed nerve will result in loss of sensibility involving the various sensory categories, i.e. light touch, pressure, pain, localization, temperature, spatial discrimination (e.g. two-point discrimination) and functional gnosis. Where the nerve lesion is in continuity, the pattern of loss can be variable, e.g. patients with a compression neuropathy may show abnormality when tested with a threshold test such as the Semmes-Weinstein monofilaments, but give a normal response to functional tests such as moving or static two-point discrimination (Callahan, 1995).

Vasomotor changes

Following complete nerve disruption, the denervated hand will be warm to the touch for the first 2 to 3 weeks due to vasodilation resulting from paralysis of the vasoconstrictors (Seddon, 1975). After this time, the hand becomes increasingly cool to the touch and readily affected by the surrounding temperature (Sunderland, 1978). Colder weather is troublesome for most patients with nerve injury.

Disruption of sympathetic nerve function affects tissue nutrition, making skin more vulnerable to injury. When injured, denervated skin usually takes longer to heal. Nail changes include ridging and furrowing, slowed growth and hardening. Atrophy of the epidermis results in decreasing prominence of the papillary ridges and there may be reduction or absence of hand sweating. Skin that is smooth and dry is said to have reduced 'tactile adhesion' (Moberg, 1962). This facility is important in preventing the slippage of objects when gripping or when performing fine manipulative tasks (Clark, 1999).

Nerve repair

The nerve is repaired as accurately as possible to facilitate the regeneration of axons down the distal connective tissue tubes. The more accurate the matching of sensory to sensory and motor to motor nerve fibres, the better is the potential reinnervation of the end organs (Fig. 5.4).

Where possible, primary repair of the nerve is undertaken. In the presence of wound contamination or associated injuries, secondary procedures are performed when conditions are more favourable, thereby giving a better result. Where there is a gap in the nerve, grafting with a suitable donor nerve (e.g. sural nerve, medial cutaneous nerve of the forearm) is undertaken to avoid tension at the

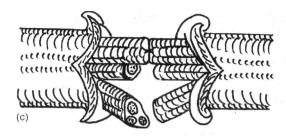
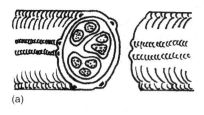
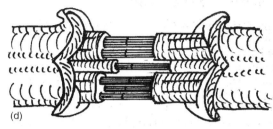
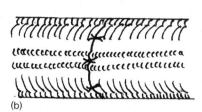

Figure 5.4. Nerve suture techniques. (a) Laceration; (b) Epineurial suture; (c) Group fascicular suture; (d) Individual fascicular suture. (Reproduced from Brushart, T. M. Nerve repair and grafting. 1999. In *Green's Operative Hand Surgery* (D. P. Green, R. N. Hotchkiss and W. C. Pederson, eds) p. 1387, Churchill Livingstone, with permission.)

repair site which will encourage proliferation of scar tissue. It is more difficult to match like axons with a nerve graft; however, because there is complete absence of tension, joint mobilization can commence earlier.

Technique

The proximal and distal nerve stumps are isolated and every attempt is made to preserve the vascular attachments. Epineurial repair is the most common technique and is used for the completely transected nerve. This is the simplest type of repair, requiring minimal magnification and a minimum number of sutures.

Perineurial (or fascicular) repair is the second most commonly used technique of nerve repair. Higher magnification is required to identify and better align the fascicular groups which should be repaired without tension. This technique allows for greater accuracy in matching fascicles of similar size. Individual fascicular repair is only rarely performed.

Healing of nerve repair

The repaired nerve sheath, whether epineurium or perineurium, takes 3 weeks to gain sufficient tensile strength to withstand stress. The repair is splinted without tension during this time.

Factors affecting nerve regeneration

Factors that can affect regeneration of nerve following injury or repair include:

1. The age of the patient (with increasing age there is a reduction in receptor populations, e.g. Meissner corpuscles).
2. The level of injury (the more proximal the lesion, the less likelihood there is of a favourable outcome).
3. Associated injuries, i.e. soft tissue loss, fractures, tendon injuries.
4. Degree of scar tissue.
5. Accuracy of fascicular alignment.

Digital nerve repair

The digital nerves are the most frequently severed peripheral nerves (Clark, 1999). To avoid tension at the repair site, digital nerve repairs are protected for three weeks with a dorsal hand-based splint that maintains the MCP joints in 50 to 70 degrees of flexion. The finger portion of the splint should allow full IP joint extension. Gentle IP joint exercises can be performed within the splint. The patient should aim for full intrinsic IP joint extension to the limit of the splint to avoid the development of a PIP joint flexion deformity.

In the case of the thumb, a small hand-based thumb post can be fitted which holds the MCP joint in 35 to 40 degrees of flexion while permitting motion at the IP joint. Following the 3-week splinting period, the patient should avoid digital hyperextension for the next 1 to 2 weeks.

Scar massage is begun following suture removal. The patient is instructed in skin care and how to avoid injury to anaesthetic skin. Desensitization exercises are performed at the repair site. Nerve regeneration is often accompanied by unpleasant paraesthesia or hyperaesthesia. A layer of Opsite Flexifix over the affected area often helps 'dampen' these unpleasant sensations (Boscheinen-Morrin and Shannon, 2000). Sensory retraining is begun when moving-touch can be perceived in the fingertip (see p. 68).

Early postoperative management following nerve repair at the wrist

After a median or ulnar nerve repair at wrist level, the hand is rested in a dorsal splint which maintains the wrist in slight flexion to avoid stress on the repair. The splint extends just beyond the tips of the fingers with the thumb remaining free. The splint is worn for 3 to 4 weeks by which time there is sufficient connective tissue strength to withstand wrist movement (Fig. 5.5).

Nerve injuries at the wrist are frequently associated with tendon injuries. In the absence of tendon injuries, gentle active finger and thumb movements can be commenced within the splint 1 to 2 days after surgery when the inflammatory response has subsided. Where there has been flexor tendon involvement, the flexor tendon protocol is used unless the surgeon advises that gentle early active movement is allowed. To minimize stress on the tendon repair, full passive finger flexion range should be established prior to the commencement of active motion.

Scar management and desensitization

Sutures are removed 10 to 14 days after surgery. Scar softening and desensitization at the repair site are commenced. Gentle oil massage should be carried out four to six times a day as part of a home programme. Initially, massage is light otherwise it cannot be tolerated due to hypersensitivity. As tolerance to touch improves, pressure is gradually increased. Extreme hypersensitivity is managed with transcutaneous electrical nerve stimulation (TENS).

Scar tissue that is dense and/or raised is managed with silicone scar gel which is applied to clean, dry, oil-free skin. The gel is also helpful in acting as a 'shock absorber' over the repaired nerve.

Patient education

Patient education is an important aspect of management following a peripheral nerve lesion. Patients should be informed of the following:

1. That muscle wasting increases in the early stages following nerve injury.
2. How to avoid injury and take care of anaesthetic skin; the patient will need to compensate visually until protective sensation has returned.
3. How to avoid deformity due to muscle imbalance by corrective splinting and maintaining mobility of joint and soft tissue structures.
4. That the average rate of nerve regeneration is approximately 1 mm per day.
5. That paraesthesia (tingling or pins and needles) and hyperaesthesia (painful hypersensitivity) are normal manifestations of nerve regeneration and will diminish with time and use of the hand.

Later stage postoperative management (4 to 6 weeks)

Gentle active wrist movements are commenced after 4 weeks. Active wrist extension is initially carried out with the fingers held flexed as there is often considerable tethering of structures, i.e. skin, nerve and tendons, resulting in soft tissue tightness.

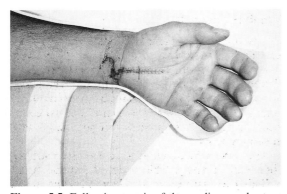

Figure 5.5. Following repair of the median or ulnar nerve at the wrist, the hand is rested in a dorsal splint which maintains the wrist in slight flexion.

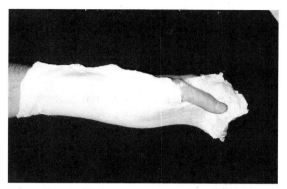

Figure 5.6. Serial plaster casts are used to overcome soft tissue tightness on the volar aspect of the wrist and/or fingers.

Overcoming soft tissue tightness

A mild flexion deformity of the wrist can be managed with a cock-up wrist splint which holds the wrist in neutral or slight extension. If the flexion deformity involves the wrist and fingers, serial extension casting is commenced between the 4th and 5th weeks. The wrist and fingers are casted in a position of correction that provides only a negligible stretch. The initial cast should hold the wrist and fingers in the position achieved by the patient when asked to actively extend to maximum range (Fig. 5.6).

This position should not cause pain and the fingertips are checked for signs of skin blanching that indicate excessive pressure. The skin, particularly areas of altered or absent sensibility, are checked regularly for signs of pressure areas. The splint is used during the night and intermittently throughout the day. Wearing time may need to be increased slowly from initial periods of 1 to 2 hours. Hand oedema is managed with a lycra pressure glove which will also exert a gentle extension force to the digits.

Tendon adherence

Due to adherence of soft tissue structures at the repair site, active movement of the fingers and thumb occurs as a 'mass' action. To promote effective tendon glide, active finger and thumb exercises should be performed individually with stabilization of more proximal joints (Fig. 5.7). The patient is advised to perform short exercise sessions on an hourly basis with at least 10 to 15 repetitions of movement. Finger movements are

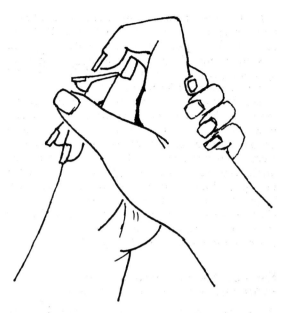

Figure 5.7. To promote tendon glide, interphalangeal joints should be exercised with stabilization of the more proximal joints.

more effectively performed when the wrist is supported in slight extension with a brace or thermoplastic splint.

Protection in cold weather

As the nerve-injured hand is vulnerable to the effects of the cold, the use of a thermal glove for protection in winter is recommended. Prior to exercise, the hand can be soaked in warm water for 10 to 15 minutes to improve comfort and mobility.

Week 6 onwards

Gentle resistance is added to flexion and extension exercises. The patient can attempt to actively extend the fingers and wrist simultaneously if flexor tightness has been overcome. Where soft tissue tightness remains, serial casting is continued until full simultaneous wrist/digital extension has been achieved. This process can sometimes take several months.

The patient is encouraged to use the hand for light daily activity. This may require functional splinting to oppose the thumb in a median nerve lesion or the use of an anti-claw splint in an ulnar nerve lesion. Where gripping is a problem, utensils can be 'built-up' with Handitube.

Care of denervated skin

Denervated skin becomes smooth, shiny, fragile and prone to injury. Skin should be nourished regularly to maintain suppleness. Apart from the potential danger of heat and sharp implements, patients should be alert to pressure areas that can arise from friction during activity or pressure areas resulting from prolonged contact of the denervated area with splints or simply resting against a hard surface. Frequently used utensils and tools can be padded to avoid these problems.

Specific nerve lesions

Median nerve

In a median nerve lesion, the hand is referred to as a 'simian' or monkey hand because of the flat appearance of the thenar musculature and the inability to rotate the thumb to oppose the digits. The thumb tends to lie beside the index finger because of the unopposed action of extensor pollicis longus and adductor pollicis (Fig. 5.8).

Low lesion

In a low lesion (i.e. at wrist level), the following muscles are affected: abductor pollicis brevis, flexor pollicis brevis and opponens pollicis (these three muscles comprise the thenar eminence) and the 1st and 2nd lumbricals.

  This results in:

1. Loss of thumb opposition.
2. Hyperextension of the MCP joints of the index and middle fingers from overaction of the extensor digitorum communis (EDC).

High lesion

A high lesion (elbow or neck) involves the following muscles in addition to the above-mentioned: flexor pollicis longus (anterior interosseous branch of median nerve), flexor digitorum profundus (FDP) to index and middle fingers (anterior interosseous branch), pronator quadratus (anterior interosseous branch), pronator teres (main branch of median nerve), flexor carpi radialis (main branch), palmaris longus (main branch) and flexor digitorum superficialis to all digits (main branch) (Fig. 5.9).

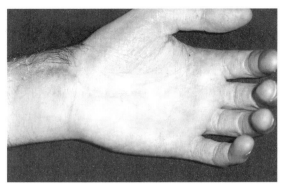

Figure 5.8. In a median nerve lesion the thenar eminence has a flat appearance and the thumb lies beside the index finger because of the unopposed action of extensor pollicis longus and abductor pollicis.

  This results in:

1. Loss of flexion to the thumb IP joint and finger flexion (other than FDP action to the ring and little fingers).
2. Loss of forearm pronation.
3. Weak radial deviation of the wrist.

The combined loss of sensibility and thumb opposition significantly affects hand function. Power grip is also affected because of the loss of the stabilizing action of the thumb. Loss of thumb palmar abduction results in an inability to grasp larger objects such as a glass.

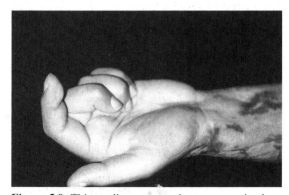

Figure 5.9. This median nerve lesion was sustained during a crush injury to the forearm. Note the anterior interosseous syndrome with loss of function of FPL and FDP to the index finger. Note also the blister on the tip of the index finger from contact with a kettle.

Trick movement

In a low-level median nerve lesion, pinch grip is achieved by the action of flexor pollicis longus and adductor pollicis against the radial side of the index finger.

Lively splint

A rotation strap made from neoprene or stretch tape (e.g. Microfoam) is used to bring the thumb into palmar abduction and opposition to facilitate pinch grip (Fig. 5.10).

Associated problems

1. Injury to skin (Fig. 5.11).
2. Contracted thumb web space; this can be overcome with serial C-splints that gently stretch the web space (Fig. 5.12).

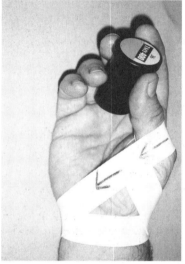

Figure 5.10. A rotation strap will elevate the thumb from its adducted posture and reposition it in opposition to the index and middle fingers.

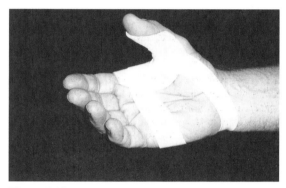

Figure 5.12. Serial C-splints are used to overcome a tight thumb web that can develop following a median nerve lesion.

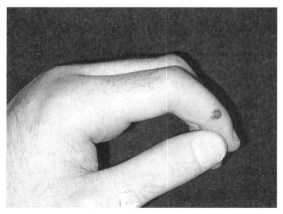

Figure 5.11. Anaesthetic skin is very vulnerable to injury from contact with hot surfaces, prolonged contact with hard surfaces or friction 'burns' during prolonged activity.

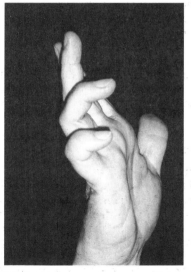

Figure 5.13. An ulnar nerve lesion results in a claw deformity of the ring and little fingers regardless of the lesion level.

Ulnar nerve

An ulnar nerve lesion results in a claw hand regardless of the level of the nerve lesion. The MCP joints of the ring and little fingers assume a position of hyperextension and IP joint flexion (Fig. 5.13).

Low lesion (wrist level)

The following muscles are affected: abductor digiti minimi, flexor digiti minimi, opponens digiti minimi (these three muscles comprise the hypo-thenar eminence); adductor pollicis, all dorsal interossei, all palmar interossei and the medial two lumbricals, i.e. the lumbricals to the ring and little fingers.

This results in:

1. Loss of finger abduction and adduction.
2. Loss of thumb adduction.
3. Clawing of the ring and little fingers – this is due to loss of the interossei and the unopposed action of extensor digitorum communis and extensor digiti minimi; this posture is known as Duchenne's sign.
4. Inability to elevate the 5th metacarpal to enable effective opposition between the thumb and little finger.

High lesion (above the elbow)

Together with the muscles involved in a low lesion, only two other muscles are affected: flexor carpi ulnaris and flexor digitorum profundus to the ring and little fingers. This results in:

1. Weakened ulnar deviation of the wrist because of unopposed action of extensor carpi ulnaris.
2. Loss of flexion at the DIP joints of the little and ring fingers; this is known as Pollock's sign.

Power grip is significantly diminished in an ulnar nerve lesion. Pinch grip is also affected through loss of the first dorsal interosseous muscle and adductor pollicis. This loss results in instability in pinching the thumb against the index finger (Froment's sign).

Trick movements

1. In the absence of adductor pollicis, adduction of the thumb to the index finger is achieved through the combined action of flexor pollicis longus and extensor pollicis longus.

2. In the absence of the 3rd and 4th lumbricals, attempts to flex the MCP joints of the ring and little fingers will result in acute flexion of the IP joints of these digits.
3. In the absence of the dorsal interossei function, finger abduction is mimicked by the digital extensors, particularly in the case of the index and little fingers which have a second extensor, i.e. extensor indicis proprius and extensor digiti minimi, respectively.
4. In the absence of volar interossei function, finger adduction is mimicked by relaxation of the digital extensors and contraction of the extrinsic finger flexors.
5. On attempting to oppose the little finger to the thumb, the IP joints of the little finger will markedly flex to compensate for the lack of 5th metacarpal elevation owing to loss of opponens digiti minimi function.

Associated problems

1. Abduction deformity of the little finger

The abductor digiti minimi is the first muscle to recover following an ulnar nerve lesion at the wrist. As recovery proceeds, the little finger becomes progressively abducted. This posture can sometimes interfere with function. To overcome this, the little finger can be buddy-strapped to the adjacent ring finger during activity.

2. Hyperaesthesia along the ulnar border of the hand

Nerve regeneration can be accompanied by hyper-sensitivity. This can be troublesome during writing. Patients are encouraged to practise desensitization exercises frequently throughout the day. Covering the affected area with a layer of Opsite Flexifix can often help to reduce sensitivity.

3. Claw deformity

This deformity can be controlled with a variety of anti-claw splints. The principle of these splints is to support the MCP joints in flexion thus allowing the long extensors to act on the IP joints in the absence of the ulnar-innervated intrinsics. This is known as Bouvier's manoeuvre (Fig. 5.14).

Radial nerve

A radial nerve lesion results in a wrist drop deformity. The wrist falls into approximately 45 degrees of flexion because the wrist flexors are unopposed by the wrist extensors. The thumb falls

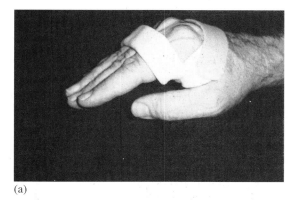
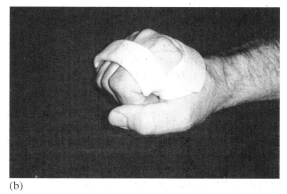

(a)   (b)

Figure 5.14. (a) The static 'spaghetti' splint controls the hyperextension deformity of the MCP joints and facilitates full interphalangeal joint extension by maintaining the MCP joints in slight flexion. (b) The splint does not hamper finger flexion and therefore allows the hand to function.

into flexion and palmar abduction because the thumb intrinsics are unopposed by abductor pollicis longus, extensor pollicis longus and extensor pollicis brevis (Fig. 5.15).

The MCP joints of the fingers fall into slight flexion because the intrinsic hand muscles, i.e. the interossei and lumbricals, are unopposed by extensor digitorum communis.

The most common site of radial nerve injury is at the radial groove of the humerus. Where this is the case, the following muscles are affected: triceps, brachioradialis, extensor carpi radialis longus, extensor carpi radialis brevis, extensor carpi ulnaris, extensor digitorum communis, extensor pollicis

longus, extensor pollicis brevis and abductor pollicis longus.

This results in loss of:

1. Elbow extension (high lesion).
2. Flexion of the elbow with the forearm in midposition (i.e. brachioradialis function).
3. Wrist extension.
4. Digital MCP joint extension.
5. Thumb extension.

Patients with a radial nerve palsy have poor grip function owing to a lack of stabilizing action of the wrist extensors.

Trick movements

1. There may appear to be contraction of the wrist extensors following strong finger and wrist flexion; this is purely due to relaxation of the flexors.
2. When the patient attempts to extend the fingers, flexion of the MCP joints will be observed due to compensatory efforts by the intrinsic muscles whose action is to flex the MCP joints and simultaneously extend the IP joints.
3. Thumb IP extension is achieved during palmar abduction owing to the accessory insertion of abductor pollicis brevis into the extensor apparatus.

Splinting

A lively radial palsy splint can restore the reciprocal tenodesis action of finger extension-wrist

Figure 5.15. This wrist drop deformity resulted from injury to the radial nerve following a crush injury. Note that the thumb has not fallen into palmar abduction because the median nerve was also affected. Note also that the MCP joints have not fallen into flexion because of skin contracture following extensive grafting.

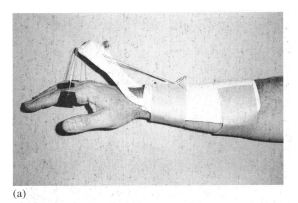
(a)

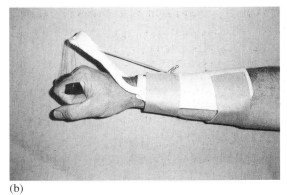
(b)

Figure 5.16. (a) In a radial nerve palsy a lively splint can restore the reciprocal tenodesis action of finger extension-wrist flexion and finger flexion-wrist extension. When the hand is relaxed, the splint maintains the wrist and fingers in neutral extension. (b) When the patient actively flexes the fingers, the wrist is brought into a functional range of extension. This splint utilizes static tension by way of nylon monofilament.

flexion and finger flexion-wrist extension. This splint employs a static suspension line (nylon thread) (Fig. 5.16).

Hand function can also be significantly enhanced with a simple cock-up wrist brace which places the wrist in 30 to 40 degrees of

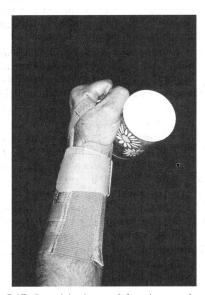

Figure 5.17. Surprisingly good function can be achieved with a simple wrist cock-up splint. The slightly extended wrist accommodates optimal function of the finger flexors and enables grasp. To release objects, sufficient digital extension is usually gained through the intrinsic musculature which extends the interphalangeal joints.

extension. Patients achieve a functional degree of digital extension using the intrinsic musculature to extend the IP joints (Fig. 5.17). It is the experience of this author that most patients reject the lively splint in favour of the static wrist brace when provided with both splints. Regardless of the type of splint used, it is important to maintain wrist support to prevent stretching of the dorsal hand structures.

Sensory retraining after median nerve repair

Patients with a sensibility deficit have the ability to adapt and compensate for this loss if they are well motivated and prepared to engage the hand in day-to-day activities (Onne, 1962). A formal sensory re-education programme can utilize learning principles such as attention, feedback, memory and reinforcement, and thereby expedite this process. These higher cortical functions, whilst not able to speed up axonal regeneration or create the formation of receptors, will help patients to interpret the altered sensory impulses that reach the brain from the peripheral nerves.

The best known of these re-education programmes are those described by Wynn Parry and Slater (1976) and Dellon et al. (1974). The aim of retraining is to improve stereognostic ability, i.e. the recognition of an object by assessing its shape, weight, size and texture. This results in improved functional dexterity even though two-point discrimination may be sub-optimal.

Timing of programme commencement

When the patient is able to discern moving-touch in the fingertips, sensory retraining is begun. Moving-touch precedes light touch which, in turn, precedes discriminative touch (Callahan, 1995). Moving-touch can be assessed with the examiner's fingertip or with Semmes-Weinstein monofilaments which should record 4.31 or lower to qualify for retraining.

Formal sensibility testing for nerve regeneration can be carried out every 6 to 8 weeks (See Chapter 1 – 'Assessment').

Treatment parameters

Sensory retraining sessions should ideally be performed four times each day. Sessions should be kept short and should take place in a quiet environment to eliminate distraction.

Localization

While the patient may be able to perceive the monofilament or fingertip, localization of the stimulus may be inaccurate. Retraining incorporates both moving- and constant-touch. Moving-touch perception returns ahead of constant-touch perception.

With the eyes closed, the stimulus is applied to the skin. The patient is then asked to identify the area with eyes opened. If localization is incorrect, the stimulus is again applied with the patient observing the manoeuvre and integrating both the visual and sensory impressions. Different areas of the palm and fingertips are then tested and retrained. Progress can be recorded on a grid pattern. Reinforcement by repetition is integral to training.

Discrimination training using textures, shapes and everyday objects

With vision occluded, the patient is asked to describe a variety of textures. These should initially be quite different to allow for easy discrimination and can include textures such as: sandpaper, sheepskin, velvet, pimple rubber, carpet, leather, towelling and silk. The patient is encouraged to describe his sensory impressions, e.g. 'rough', 'smooth', 'prickly' or 'spongy', as this description will often help the patient deduce the texture. In this way, the patient is reproducing

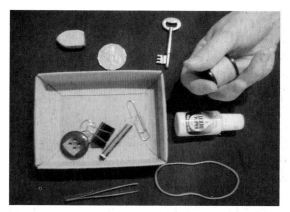

Figure 5.18. The final stage of sensory retraining involves trying to identify everyday objects.

in slow motion what the normal hand does automatically and with great speed. Where distinction is poor or inaccurate, the patient moves the texture over the affected area again while watching the manoeuvre so that the tactile-visual image can be reinforced.

The process is then repeated using different shaped blocks. Larger sizes are used initially. The patient is encouraged to slowly move the blocks in the hand, thereby gaining impressions of smooth surfaces and corners. When these have been mastered, the patient progresses to smaller sizes.

The final stage of retraining involves the use of everyday objects. Larger objects are used before smaller objects are introduced. The types of objects used in testing and training should reflect the everyday experience of the patient. Again, the patient is encouraged to explore the object slowly, gleaning information regarding its size, shape, density, temperature and texture. More textures and objects are added to the programme as the patient demonstrates progress (Fig. 5.18).

Retraining sessions can be curtailed when the patient has attained the desired level of functional dexterity. The maintenance of this dexterity, however, relies on the hand being engaged in daily use so that the training effect is not lost.

References

Boscheinen-Morrin, J. and Shannon, J. (2000). Opsite Flexifix: an effective adjunct in the management of pain and hypersensitivity in the hand. *Aust. Occup. Ther. J.,* (submitted for publication September, 2000).

Bowden, R. E. M. and Gutmann, E. (1944). Denervation and reinnervation of human voluntary muscle. *Brain*, **67**, 273–313.

Callahan, A. D. (1995). Sensibility assessment: prerequisites and techniques for nerve lesions in continuity and nerve lacerations. In *Rehabilitation of the Hand: Surgery and Therapy* (J. M. Hunter, E. J. Mackin and A. D. Callahan, eds) pp. 129–52, Mosby.

Clark, T. (1999). Digital nerve repair: The relationship between sensibility and dexterity. Thesis. (MSc – coursework). Curtin University of Technology, Perth, Australia.

Dellon, A. L., Curtis, R. M. and Edgerton, M. T. (1974). Re-education of sensation in the hand after nerve injury and repair. *Plast. Reconstr. Surg.*, **53**, 297–305.

Lundborg, G. (1975). Structure and function of the intraneural microvessels as related to trauma, edema formation and nerve function. *J. Bone Joint Surg.*, **57A**, 938.

Lundborg, G. (1988). *Nerve Injury and Repair.* Churchill Livingstone.

Moberg, E. (1962). Criticism and study of methods for examining sensibility in the hand. *Neurology*, **12**, 8–19.

Onne, L. (1962). Recovery of sensibility and sudomotor activity in the hand after nerve suture. *Acta Chir. Scand. (Suppl.)* **300**, 1–69.

Seddon, H. J. (1975). *Surgical Disorders of the Peripheral Nerves.* Churchill Livingstone.

Stoll, G., Griffin, J. W., Li, C. Y. and Trapp, B. D. (1989). Wallerian degeneration in the peripheral nervous system: participation of both Schwann cells and macrophages in myelin degradation. *J. Neurocytol.*, **18**, 671–83.

Sunderland, S. (1978). *Nerves and Nerve Injuries.* Churchill Livingstone.

Sunderland, S. and Bradley, K. C. (1949). The cross-sectional area of peripheral nerve trunks devoted to nerve fibers. *Brain*, **72**, 428–49.

Weiss, D. G. and Gorio, A. (eds) (1982). *Axoplasmic Transport in Physiology and Pathology.* Springer-Verlag.

Wynn Parry, C. B. and Salter, M. (1976). Sensory re-education after median nerve lesions. *Hand*, **8**, 250–7.

Further reading

Bell-Krotoski, J. (1995). Sensibility testing: current concepts. In *Rehabilitation of the Hand: Surgery and Therapy* (J. M. Hunter, E. J. Mackin and A. D. Callahan, eds) pp. 109–28, Mosby.

Birch, R. and Raji, A. R. M. (1991). Repair of median and ulnar nerves. Primary suture is best. *J. Bone Joint Surg.*, **73B**, 154–7.

Brushart, T. M. (1994). Peripheral nerve regeneration: strategies to augment specificity. *Adv. Operat. Orthop. 2(Suppl.)*, **20**.

Brushart, T. M. (1999). Nerve repair and grafting. In *Green's Operative Hand Surgery* (D. P. Green, R. N. Hotchkiss and W. C. Pederson, eds) pp. 1381–403, Churchill Livingstone.

Butler, D. S. (1991). *Mobilisation of the Nervous System.* Churchill Livingstone.

Chassard, M., Pham, E. and Comtet, J. J. (1993). Two-point discrimination tests versus functional sensory recovery in both median and ulnar nerve complete transections. *J. Hand Surg.*, **18B**, 790–6.

Colditz, J. C. (1995). Splinting the hand with a peripheral nerve injury. In *Rehabilitation of the Hand: Surgery and Therapy* (J. M. Hunter, E. J. Mackin and A. D. Callahan, eds) pp. 679–92, Mosby.

Conolly, W. B. and Morrin, J. (1981). Sensory rehabilitation in the hand. *Lancet*, **i**, 135.

Curtis, R. M. and Dellon, A. L. (1980). Sensory re-education after peripheral nerve injury. In *Management of Peripheral Nerve Injuries* (G. Omer and M. Spinner, eds) pp. 769–78, W. B. Saunders.

Dellon, A. L. Reinnervation of denervated Meissner corpuscles: a sequential histologic study in the monkey following fascicular repair. *J. Hand Surg.*, **1**, 98.

Dellon, A. L. and Jabaley, M. E. (1982). Re-education of sensation in the hand following nerve suture. *Clin. Orthop.*, **163**, 75.

Efstathopoulos, D., Gerostathopoulos, N., Misitzis, et al. (1995). Clinical assessment of primary digital nerve repair. *Acta Orthop. Scand. Suppl.*, **264**, 45–7.

Jerosch-Herold, C. (1993). Measuring outcome in median nerve injuries. *J. Hand Surg.*, **18B**, 624–8.

Kallio, P. K. and Vastamaeki, M. (1993). An analysis of the results of late reconstruction of 132 median nerves. *J. Hand Surg.*, **18B**, 97–105.

Kendall, F. P. (1983). *Muscles – Testing and Function.* Williams & Wilkins.

Lundborg, G. (1993). Peripheral nerve injuries: pathophysiology and strategies for treatment. *J. Hand Ther.*, **6**, 179.

Millesi, H. (1985). Peripheral nerve repair. Terminology, questions and facts. *J. Reconstr. Microsurg.*, **2**, 21–31.

Moran, C. A. and Callahan, A. D. (1986). Sensibility measurement and management. In *Hand Rehabilitation (Clinics in Physical Therapy Series)* (C. A. Moran, ed.) pp. 45–68, Churchill Livingstone.

Smith, K. L. (1995). Nerve response to injury and repair. In *Rehabilitation of the Hand: Surgery and Therapy* (J. M. Hunter, E. J. Mackin and A. D. Callahan, eds) pp. 609–626, Mosby.

Sunderland, S. (1990). The anatomy and physiology of nerve injury. *Muscle Nerve*, **13**, 771–84.

6

Tendon transfers

Where muscle function has been lost through injury or disease, hand function can be improved by the transfer of an expendable muscle-tendon unit with the aim of restoring balance to the hand. Selected early transfers can optimize sensibility re-education when performed in the dominant hand (Citron and Taylor, 1987).

Prerequisites for tendon transfer

1. The patient must be a suitable candidate for reconstructive surgery.
2. All joints that will be affected either directly or indirectly by the transfer must be fully passively mobile as transferred tendons cannot move or correct stiffened or contracted joints.
3. All skin and soft tissue in the vicinity of the transfer must be pliable and mobile. Any pre-existing soft tissue adherence will prevent effective tendon glide of the transferred tendon. Also, any soft tissue tightness, e.g. a contracted thumb web, will require correction prior to surgery.
4. The muscle-tendon unit to be transferred must be sufficiently strong to perform its new function in its altered position.

Contraindications

1. Contracture of joints or skin that would limit movement.
2. Lack of a suitable muscle or muscles for transfer.

3. A progressive neuropathy, e.g. nerve damage following radiation therapy.
4. Complicating medical conditions, e.g. muscle spasm or circulatory inadequacy.

Preoperative preparation

A full muscle assessment of the arm is undertaken to determine precisely which muscles are affected and to ascertain which muscles can be used for transfer. A muscle-strengthening programme is devised for the patient to carry out independently so that motivation and commitment to therapy can be evaluated (Warren, 1997).

All surgical stages must be planned prior to the first procedure. When choosing transfers, it is important to know the strength of the muscle and its excursion. The strength of a muscle is proportional to its cross-sectional area and is expressed as a tension fraction. The excursion of a muscle is determined by the length of its fibres. Because this is constantly changing, the resting fibre length is recorded. These measurements have been determined by Brand et al. (1981) and abstracts from their charts are given in the table below.

Surgical considerations

Choice of transfer tendon

The retraining of muscle function following transfer is easier when there is synergism between the muscle's original function and its new action

Table 6.1. Alphabetic list of the main muscles of the forearm with resting fibre length and tension fraction

Muscle	Resting fibre length (cm)	Tension fraction (%)
Abductor digiti minimi	4.0	1.4
Abductor pollicis brevis	3.7	1.1
Abductor pollicis longus	4.6	3.1
Brachioradialis	16.1 (average)	2.4
Extensor carpi radialis brevis	6.1	4.2
Extensor carpi radialis longus	9.3	3.5
Extensor carpi ulnaris	4.5	4.5
Extensor digitorum communis	5.6 (average)	1.4
Extensor digiti minimi	5.9	1.0
Extensor indicis proprius	5.5	1.0
Extensor pollicis brevis	4.3	0.8
Extensor pollicis longus	5.7	1.3
Flexor carpi radialis	5.2	4.1
Flexor carpi ulnaris	4.2	6.7
Flexor digitorum profundus	6.5 (average)	2.9
Flexor digitorum superficialis	7.1 (average)	2.1
Flexor pollicis brevis	3.6	1.3
Flexor pollicis longus	5.9	2.7
Opponens pollicis	2.4	1.9
Palmaris longus	5.0	1.0
Pronator teres	5.1	5.5

(Davis and Barton, 1999). The use of superficialis tendons may be an exception to this because there is more independent cortical control compared to other muscles in the hand (Green, 1999).

Expendability of the donor

The removal of a tendon for transfer should not leave an unacceptable loss of function, e.g. only one of the two main wrist flexors (i.e. FCR or FCU) should be used as palmaris longus is an inadequate substitute for their loss.

Incision sites

The suturing of skin directly over tendon sutures should be avoided, as should incisions along the new line of the transferred tendon.

The transfer pathway

The most efficient transfer is one that passes in a direct line from its origin to the insertion of the tendon that it is substituting. If the transfer cannot perform its new function with a straight line of

pull, it should pass through no more than one pulley. Acute angulation of the transfer at the pulley should be avoided.

Where possible, natural 'tracks' should be used. If a new one is needed, there should be no force used when tunneling through tissues such as scar, fascia or muscle. Tunnels need to be wide enough to permit free passage of the tendon. If passage through a sheet of fascia is necessary, there should be sufficient excision to minimize obstructing adhesions. The creation of a tunnel by force is likely to result in adhesions.

Single or dual insertion techniques

Tendon transfers are most efficient when they perform only one active function. The effectiveness of a tendon transfer is reduced when it is expected to produce two dissimilar functions even when they are not directly opposed (Green, 1999).

Tension of transfers

The proper tension in a transfer is critical to the outcome of the procedure. For some transfer procedures, e.g. the standard thumb opponens replacement, tensions have been determined. For others, tension must be carefully estimated and a certain level of experience is necessary before the surgeon develops the 'feel' for proper tension. Most tendon junctions stretch in the first three months and it is better to err on the side of slightly too much tension than not enough.

Tendon junctions

Where grafts are used to extend tendons or where there are mid-tendon junctions, tidy suturing is required. Loose tendon ends, long threads, prominent knots or potentially irritating non-absorbable sutures, e.g. silk, should not be left exposed as they may irritate and/or cause adhesions.

Healing times

The repair is either tendon to tendon or tendon to bone and requires about 4 weeks of healing before it is safe to subject it to the stress of active movement. Healing also occurs along the course of the transferred tendon and can result in adhesions to surrounding tissues.

Opponensplasty for median nerve palsy

Abductor pollicis brevis is the prime muscle of thumb opposition. Some opposition is also produced by opponens pollicis and flexor pollicis brevis (Cooney and Linscheid, 1984). Following a complete lesion of the median nerve, thumb abduction and opposition are frequently retained because of the variability of thenar muscle innervation. The flexor pollicis brevis muscle frequently has dual median and ulnar nerve innervation (Rowntree, 1949).

The success of opponensplasty will be determined by the quality of sensibility. In the case of a high median nerve lesion in adults, sensory recovery is usually poor and the benefit of this procedure is doubtful.

Requirements prior to opponensplasty for low level lesion (wrist)

1. Normal or maximal thumb web span.
2. Mobile thumb joints.
3. Full mobility of the unaffected digits.

4. Supple skin so that the tendon transfer is not limited by subdermal scarring.

The basic requirements for restoring thumb opposition were established by Bunnell (1938) who identified the pisiform as the best location for a fixed pulley because this keeps the transfer in line with the abductor pollicis brevis muscle.

Opponensplasty using superficialis of the ring finger

Technique

The superficialis tendon of the ring finger is harvested through an incision in the distal palm to avoid injury to the flexor sheath at the level of the PIP joint. Where patients exhibit joint hypermobility, tenodesis of the PIP joint is performed to prevent a secondary hyperextension deformity.

About 3–4 cm proximal to the wrist, a flap is raised using the anterior half of the flexor carpi ulnaris tendon. The flap is elevated as far as 1 cm proximal to the tendon's insertion into the pisiform. It is then fashioned into a loop with a 1 cm central diameter and serves as a pulley (Bunnell, 1938). To prevent migration of the pulley, the

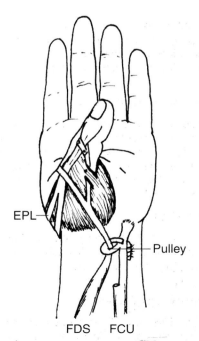

Figure 6.1. Opponensplasty for low median nerve palsy using FDS of the ring finger as motor.

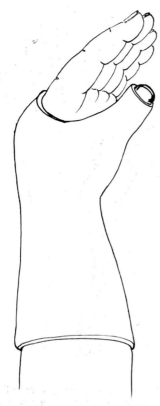

Figure 6.2. The position of immobilization following opponensplasty has the wrist in neutral extension and the thumb in full opposition with the IP joint held in extension.

distally based slip of FCU can be attached to the tendon of extensor carpi ulnaris (Sakellarides, 1970) (Fig. 6.1).

The flexor retinaculum and ulnar border of the palmar aponeurosis can provide an alternative pulley to the one described (Thompson–Royle transfer, 1942). The superficialis tendon is divided into two slips. One slip is attached as far distally as possible to the abductor pollicis brevis tendon and the other, more distally, into the extensor apparatus.

Postoperative management

The wrist is immobilized in neutral extension with the thumb held in full opposition and the IP joint of the thumb held in extension to protect the attachment to the extensor mechanism (Fig. 6.2). The fingers are left free to move. If the PIP joint has

been tenodesed to prevent hyperextension deformity, it should be splinted in about 45 degrees of flexion during the immobilization period.

Weeks 0 to 4

During the first 3 to 4 postoperative weeks, the transfer is completely immobilized to protect the tendon junctions. Gentle active finger movements can be performed. If the postoperative plaster is comfortable and maintains the correct position, it need not be replaced. During this period, however, the splint should be checked regularly to ensure that it is comfortable and that the correct position is being maintained.

Weeks 4 to 6

The hand is taken out of the splint and active use of the transferred tendon is commenced. Throughout this fortnight, the splint is worn between exercise sessions and during sleep. With the wrist held in mild flexion and the other digits trapped in extension, the patient is asked to flex the donor finger, i.e. the ring finger. This action should produce some thumb abduction and opposition. If this is not occurring, it may be necessary to slightly 'straighten' the wrist so that a little tension is placed on the transfer to help facilitate its action. This action is repeated until the patient is able to demonstrate spontaneous movement of the thumb.

To help facilitate this spontaneity, the patient can be asked to touch the thumb to the little finger or to pick up a light object. Non-resistive activity, such as playing board games, should be encouraged. As sensory recovery may still be suboptimal, the game pieces should not be too small and can be covered with a textured fabric to enhance grip. Exercise and activity sessions are kept short at this stage to avoid fatigue of the transferred muscle. The patient should perform 6 daily sessions with each session lasting between 5 and 10 minutes (Stanley, 1995).

From the 5th week onward, active abduction and opposition are practised with the hand in all positions. It is important to emphasize wrist movements as these alternately relax and tighten the opponensplasty (Davis and Barton, 1999). If the patient is overusing flexor pollicis longus during active exercise, the thumb IP joint can be immobilized in extension with a small thermoplastic splint to isolate the action of the transfer.

Scar softening is an important part of the home programme during this time. Oil massage along the scar line should be carried out 4 to 6 times daily. Silicone gel is used at night and in between exercise sessions.

Week 6 onwards

Graded resistance is applied to the transferred tendon by way of exercise and activity. Massage and pressure therapy are continued until scar resolution has been achieved. The transfer should be able to withstand normal loading 12 to 14 weeks after surgery.

Alternative procedures

1. Extensor indicis proprius opponensplasty

This transfer has an advantage over the superficialis transfer in that it does not compromise gross grip strength through the loss of a digital flexor (Burkhalter et al., 1973). The ulnar border of the wrist is used as a natural pulley and the transfer is inserted into the tendon of abductor pollicis brevis.

Because extensor indicis proprius has a relatively short excursion, the wrist should be immobilized in 30 degrees of flexion so as to relax the transfer during the immobilization period (Davis and Barton, 1999).

2. Camitz palmaris longus opponensplasty

This procedure is used for patients with a functional disability related to severe carpal tunnel syndrome and can be performed at the same time as carpal tunnel release. The palmaris longus transfer is usually attached to the insertion of abductor pollicis brevis (Terrono et al., 1993) and restores palmar abduction rather than opposition (Fig. 6.3).

The wrist is maintained in neutral extension with the thumb in opposition and the MCP joint in extension. The splint is maintained for 4 weeks and formal therapy is rarely required following this procedure.

3. Less commonly used transfers

These include: abductor digiti minimi (Huber), extensor carpi ulnaris, extensor carpi radialis longus and extensor digiti minimi.

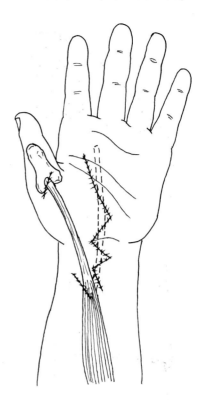

Figure 6.3. The Camitz opponensplasty utilizes the palmaris longus tendon which is lengthened with a strip of palmar aponeurosis and attached to the abductor pollicis brevis insertion. (Reproduced from Davis, T. R. C. and Barton, N. J. Median nerve palsy. 1999. In *Green's Operative Hand Surgery* (D. P. Green, R. N. Hotchkiss and W. C. Pederson, eds) p. 1509, Churchill Livingstone, with permission.)

Ulnar nerve palsy

The classic ulnar claw deformity is not always apparent following injury to this nerve. There can be several anomalous neural patterns of the ulnar nerve in the forearm and hand. This may result in all of the lumbricals being innervated by the median nerve in which case there would be no clawing of the digits.

In 50 per cent of upper limbs, there is dual innervation to the third lumbrical and this would result in clawing of the little finger only in a low level palsy. In 10 per cent of hands, the median nerve partially or completely innervates the first dorsal interosseous muscle with rare innervation by the radial nerve also occurring (Kaplan and Spinner, 1980).

Preoperative requirements for low level ulnar nerve lesion

1. The PIP joints must be fully mobile in passive extension and the MCP joints fully mobile in passive flexion.
2. Soft tissues should be free of contracting scar and have adequate circulation.

Available donors

Tendon transfers in an ulnar nerve palsy aim to restore flexion of the MCP joints and thumb adduction. Almost any tendon that crosses the wrist can be used. Suitable muscle-tendon units include: flexor digitorum superficialis, extensor carpi radialis longus, extensor carpi radialis brevis, flexor carpi radialis, brachioradialis and palmaris longus. The smaller extensors, i.e. extensor indicis proprius and extensor digiti minimi (quinti) can provide intrinsic function with the transfer of a muscle to two fingers each (original Fowler technique) (Fig. 6.4).

Superficialis transfers are designed to integrate MCP joint and IP joint motion. They do not, however, result in increased grip strength (Hastings and McCollam, 1994). The use of a wrist extensor to flex the MCP joints will improve gross power grip.

Intrinsic transfer using extensor carpi radialis longus

The extensor carpi radialis longus tendon is lengthened with a free tendon graft using palmaris longus (or plantaris). The graft is split into two slips that are passed through the intermetacarpal spaces between the long/ring and ring/little fingers respectively (Fig. 6.5).

Each slip is then passed volar to the deep transverse metacarpal ligament and inserted into a drill hole, on the radial aspect of the proximal phalanges of the ring and little fingers. Many surgeons transfer to all four fingers.

Postoperative management

The hand is splinted in the following position:

1. Wrist in 45 degrees of extension.
2. MCP joints in 70 degrees of flexion.
3. IP joints in full extension.
4. The thumb remains free (Fig. 6.6).

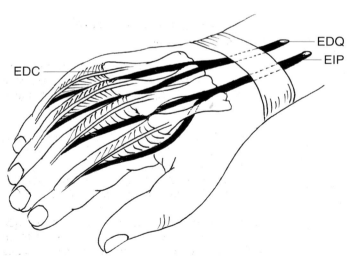

Figure 6.4. The Fowler transfer for ulnar nerve palsy uses the EIP and EDQ (or EDM) tendons, each divided into two slips.

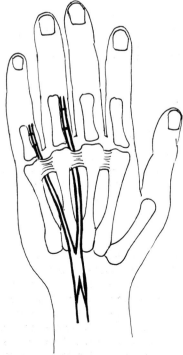

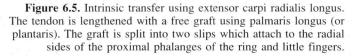

Figure 6.5. Intrinsic transfer using extensor carpi radialis longus. The tendon is lengthened with a free graft using palmaris longus (or plantaris). The graft is split into two slips which attach to the radial sides of the proximal phalanges of the ring and little fingers.

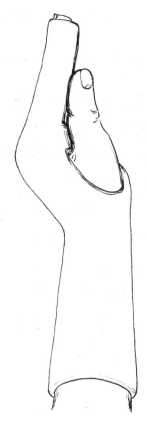

Figure 6.6. The position of immobilization following intrinsic transfer using ECRL is as follows: wrist in 45 degrees of extension, MCP joints in 70 degrees of flexion, IP joints in full extension and the thumb remaining free.

Weeks 0 to 4

The hand and forearm are maintained in the described position for the first postoperative month. If postoperative swelling has been significant, it may be necessary to change the cast after several days so that the position of immobilization is not lost.

Weeks 4 to 6

When the hand is removed from the splint and placed on the table, there will be a slight relaxation of the positions of wrist extension and MCP joint flexion. To prevent further extension of the MCP joints, the therapist places light pressure over the PIP joints. The patient is then asked to actively extend the wrist which should result in some MCP joint flexion. Extension of the IP joints should be

maintained during this manoeuvre. The hand is returned to the splint after each exercise session until the end of the 6th week.

The patient should perform this exercise on a 1 to 2 hourly basis with 5 to 10 repetitions during the 1st week of active exercise. By the 2nd week, the patient learns to localize the action of MCP joint flexion without having to extend the wrist and practises the movement with the hand in all positions, i.e. palm up and with the hand on the side.

By the 5th week, emphasis is placed on active flexion and extension of the fingers while maintaining MCP joint flexion. Gentle active wrist flexion is also begun.

Weeks 6 to 12

Light gripping activities are commenced. If active finger flexion is incomplete, the handles of everyday utensils, e.g. cutlery, can be temporarily enlarged to encourage function.

Graded resistance is applied to MCP joint flexion with the IP joints extended, i.e. intrinsic flexion. The activity programme is upgraded to restore maximum power grip. Workers involved in manual work can return to employment after the 14th week.

Alternative dynamic procedure

Superficialis transfer

The superficialis tendon of the middle (long) or ring finger is divided into 2 slips (for the ring/little fingers only) or 4 slips for all digits. Each slip is attached in one of three ways (Fig. 6.7):

1. To the lateral band of the dorsal apparatus (this insertion is associated with a high incidence of swan-neck deformity).
2. Into the A1 or A2 pulley of the flexor sheath.
3. Into a drill hole in the proximal phalanx.

The position of immobilization is: wrist in slight flexion (15 to 20 degrees), MCP flexion of 60 to 70 degrees and full extension of the IP joints (Fig. 6.8).

Static procedures

1. Capsulodesis of the MCP joints

A short flap of the MCP joint volar plate is drawn proximally and sutured into the neck of the metacarpal, thereby holding the MCP joints in 20

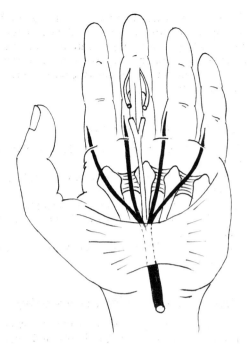

Figure 6.7. The superficialis transfer for ulnar nerve palsy using the FDS tendon of the middle (long) or ring finger. The tendon is hatched back to the level of the flexor retinaculum and divided into four slips (coloured black) which are rerouted volar to the deep transverse metacarpal ligament. The slips are attached either to the lateral band of the dorsal apparatus, into the A1 or A2 pulley or into a drill hole in the proximal phalanx.

degrees of flexion (Zancolli, 1957). Postoperatively, this position must be maintained for at least 6 weeks.

2. Flexor pulley advancement (Bunnell, 1942)

The A2 pulley is split on each side for 1.5 to 2.5 cm to the middle of the proximal phalanx. This results in 'bowstringing' of the flexors, thereby increasing movement across the MCP joint.

3. Static tenodesis

A free tendon graft (e.g., ECRL, ECU) is passed from the lateral band of the dorsal extensor apparatus to the deep transverse metacarpal ligament in the palm where it is sutured with the MCP joint in 45 degrees of flexion. Each grafted finger functions independently (Parkes, 1973).

The thumb in ulnar nerve palsy

Patients with ulnar nerve palsy lose 75 to 80 per cent of pinch grip power (Mannerfelt, 1966). The adduction force in key pinch comes primarily from adductor pollicis and the radial head of the first dorsal interosseous muscle (Omer, 1999). Restoration of pinch grip power following tendon transfer ranges between 25 and 50 per cent of normal.

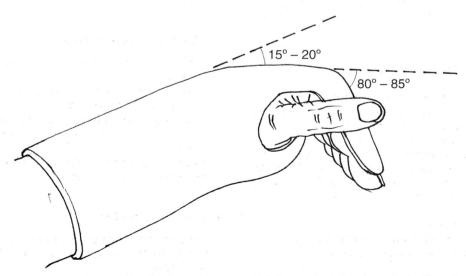

Figure 6.8. The position of immobilization following a superficialis transfer holds the wrist in slight flexion because of the flexor route of the transfer.

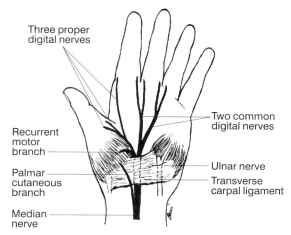

Three proper
digital nerves

Recurrent
motor
branch

Palmar
cutaneous
branch

Median
nerve

Two common
digital nerves

Ulnar nerve

Transverse
carpal ligament

Figure 7.2. The transverse carpal ligament is a thick fibrous sheet attached ulnarly to the pisiform and hook of hamate, and radially, to the scaphoid tubercle and beak of trapezium. The median nerve lies directly beneath the TCL and normally divides into six branches at the distal edge of this ligament.

1. The recurrent motor branch.
2. Three proper digital nerves (two to the thumb and one to the index finger).
3. Two common digital nerves (one to index/ middle and one to middle/ring) (Fig. 7.2).

Median nerve anomalies are common, e.g. the motor branch may be extraligamentous, transligamentous or subligamentous and may arise from the volar, radial or ulnar side of the median nerve. The most common pattern of the motor branch is extraligamentous and recurrent. Variations in the palmar cutaneous branch are also common (Siegel et al., 1993).

There are also variations in the course of the median nerve itself. It occasionally has a high or low division into its various branches and there may be a persisting median artery.

Patient presentation

The patient usually presents with numbness, pain and paraesthesia in the median nerve distribution of the hand. Because of communication between the median and ulnar nerves, symptoms may also involve the ring and little fingers. There is often associated clumsiness and weakness of pinch. Sensory changes, both subjective and objective,

usually precede weakness and wasting by weeks or months.

Characteristically, pain and paraesthesia are most distressing at night. This is related to vascular stasis caused by inactivity and pressure on the median nerve from wrist flexion or lying on the arm. The painful burning, numbness or tingling sensations may radiate up the arm to the shoulder or neck where there may be restriction to longitudinal glide of the nerve. The fingers may feel swollen and the whole arm heavy. The patient usually attempts to relieve these symptoms by hanging the arm over the side of the bed or shaking the hand. This is referred to as 'waking numbness'.

Clinical assessment

Two commonly used provocative tests to help in the clinical diagnosis of CTS are Phalen's test and Tinel's sign. While these tests are not absolutely diagnostic, they are positive in about two-thirds of patients with this syndrome.

1. Phalen's test (wrist flexion test)

This test is performed with the patient holding the forearm vertically in the air and allowing the wrist

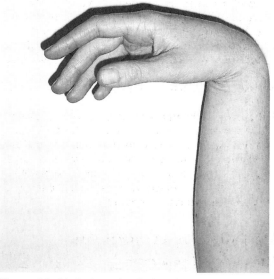

Figure 7.3. Phalen's (wrist flexion) test is performed with the forearm held vertically in the air while maintaining the wrist in flexion for a period of 60 seconds.

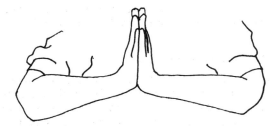

Figure 7.4. The reverse Phalen's test places the median nerve on the stretch and may elicit a positive response when the wrist flexion test is negative.

to fall into full flexion. The fingers and thumb remain relaxed. This position is held for 60 s and is considered positive if numbness and paraesthesia are elicited during this time (Fig. 7.3).

The reverse Phalen's test may be positive when the wrist flexion test is negative. The palms of the hands are placed together with the elbows raised, thus extending the wrists and placing the median nerve on the stretch (Fig. 7.4).

2. Tinel's sign

The Tinel's manoeuvre involves gentle tapping over the median nerve at wrist level. Again, if this produces symptoms, the test is considered to be positive.

3. Semmes–Weinstein monofilaments

Sensory impairment, which is not always present in CTS, can be assessed with monofilaments which may detect loss of light touch or, in more established cases, loss of protective sensation.

4. Assessment of motor function

Abnormal motor signs include weakness of the thenar muscles, especially abductor pollicis brevis. This can be tested by forcible tip-to-tip pinch between the thumb and ring finger. Weakness of lumbrical action to the middle finger may occasionally be seen.

5. Autonomic findings

As the median nerve transmits most of the sympathetic nerve supply to the hand, there may also be abnormal autonomic findings. These may include: discoloration of the skin, disorder of sweating in the hand and fingers or nail changes such as fragility, brittleness or shedding.

Causes of carpal tunnel syndrome

The causes of CTS are many and varied. Metabolic and endocrinal causes can include: pregnancy, menopause, Raynaud's disease, rheumatoid disease, diabetes, myxoedema and acromegaly. There can be an acute onset of CTS following wrist trauma, infection within the tunnel, thrombosis of an anomalous median artery or iatrogenic injection injury of the median nerve.

Occupational factors can include repetitive force (particularly where fingers and wrist are flexed simultaneously), posture, vibration and temperature of work environment.

Lifestyle factors are also believed to play an important role in the incidence of CTS. These factors include: obesity (Nathan et al., 1992), excessive alcohol consumption and tobacco use.

There is an ischaemic factor in many compression neuropathies (Gelberman and Szabo, 1986). The reduced epineurial blood flow leads to impaired axonal transport. Whilst these effects can be reversed in the early stages, prolonged endoneurial swelling with resultant fibrosis can result in permanent sensory and motor loss.

Stages of compression

1. Early

These patients have a history of recent onset and intermittent symptoms of numbness and paraesthesia. This category of patients shows the best response to conservative treatment measures which include:

1. Wrist splinting in neutral or slight extension (the carpal tunnel has maximum capacity in these positions).
2. Corticosteroid injection into the carpal tunnel (this helps reduce inflammatory oedema around the nerve).
3. Nerve gliding exercises.
4. Postural assessment in relation to the work environment or leisure activities.
5. Modification of work practices and work environment where indicated.

Wrist splinting

The wrist support is used only at night if there are no day symptoms. Intermittent day use is recommended for patients whose symptoms are also present during the day. For patients who have had

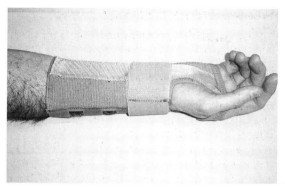

Figure 7.5. Early symptoms of CTS are managed with conservative measures that include a wrist splint to maintain the wrist in neutral or slight extension.

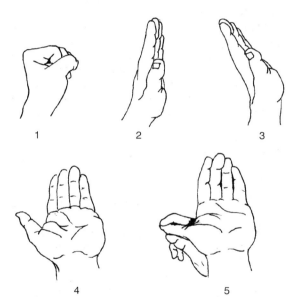

Figure 7.6. Median nerve gliding exercises can be performed as part of a conservative treatment programme or following open or endoscopic carpal tunnel decompression. Position 1: the forearm is in neutral rotation, the wrist in neutral extension and the fingers and thumb are flexed. Position 2: the wrist remains in neutral, the fingers extend and the thumb lies in neutral beside the index finger. Position 3: while the thumb remains in the neutral position, the wrist is extended while finger extension is maintained. Position 4: the wrist is returned to neutral extension and with the fingers and thumb also in neutral extension, the forearm is supinated. Position 5: with the forearm still in supination, a gentle stretch is applied to the thumb. (Redrawn with permission from Totten, P. A. and Hunter, J. M. 1991. Therapeutic techniques to enhance nerve gliding in the thoracic outlet and carpal tunnel syndromes. *Hand Clin.*, **7(3)**, 505.)

a corticosteroid injection, the wrist is rested continuously for a period of 2 weeks (Fig. 7.5).

Nerve gliding exercises

Totten and Hunter (1991) have developed a series of nerve gliding exercises for the brachial plexus and the median nerve at the carpal tunnel. A study by Wilgis and Murphy (1986) on the longitudinal excursion of peripheral nerves, determined that the greatest excursion occurred proximal to the carpal tunnel at the wrist.

The median nerve gliding exercises can be used for conservative management of CTS or post-operatively, to minimize nerve-tendon adhesions. The exercises can be performed with the patient sitting or lying supine. The head is in the midline position, the shoulder is adducted and the elbow is flexed to 90 degrees (Fig. 7.6).

The exercise sequence is performed in a slow, methodical manner with 5 to 10 repetitions every 1 to 2 hours. The manoeuvre is performed to the point where slight tension is produced, this usually manifesting as a slight pull or some change to sensibility. When this point is reached, the patient is asked to back off slightly to ease these symptoms. Some trial and error is usually necessary to establish the appropriate level of exercise. It is preferable to 'underperform' the exercises rather than to perform them too vigorously and exacerbate symptoms. Symptoms of tingling, numbness or pain following the gliding exercises should not take more than a few hours to resolve.

Brachial plexus gliding exercises

These gliding exercises address the entire length of the nerves, from proximal to distal. This manoeuvre is far more likely to produce an irritable response and should therefore be performed very cautiously. Symptoms are often not evident for several hours after the exercise and, as with the above exercises, should resolve after several hours (Fig. 7.7).

Gentle brachial plexus gliding exercises can be used in the workplace as part of a prevention/treatment strategy that also incorporates assessment/modification of postural and work habits.

2. Intermediate

Patients in this category report almost constant numbness and paraesthesia and are candidates for nerve decompression.

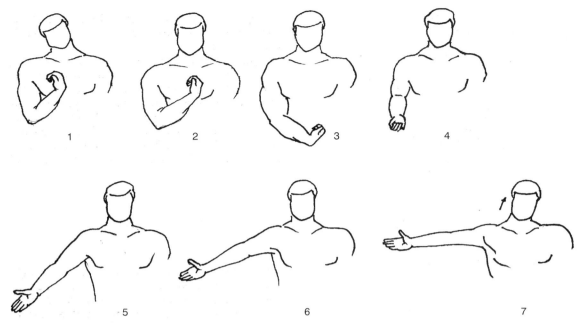

Figure 7.7. The brachial plexus programme is as follows: Position 1: the head is laterally flexed to the affected side with the elbow, wrist and fingers of the affected side in flexion. Position 2: the head comes to the neutral position. Position 3: the hand is moved across the chest and down to the hip level. Position 4: the patient gradually extends the elbow and increasingly abducts the shoulder into positions 5 and 6. Position 7: Lateral cervical flexion to the opposite side is the final component of this manoeuvre. (Redrawn with permission from Totten, P. A. and Hunter, J. M. 1991. Therapeutic techniques to enhance nerve gliding in thoracic outlet and carpal tunnel syndromes. *Hand Clin.,* **7(3)**, 505.)

3. Late

These patients have usually had longstanding symptoms. Even after decompression, there may be permanent sensory impairment and thenar wasting because of the degree of neural fibrosis. Where appropriate, these patients are offered an opposition transfer to enhance pinch grip function.

Surgery

Surgery to decompress the tunnel is indicated where conservative measures have failed to relieve symptoms. The aim of surgery is to increase the dimensions of the carpal tunnel by releasing the transverse carpal ligament and its fascial extensions.

Studies have shown that the average increase in volume of the tunnel following decompression is 24 per cent and that the tunnel is converted from an oval to a circular shape (Richman et al., 1989).

1. Open decompression

Decompression of the carpal tunnel has traditionally been performed as an open procedure. The obvious advantage of the open technique is good visualization which allows identification of anatomical anomalies. This means a reduced risk of iatrogenic injury.

The skin incision is made 2–3 mm ulnar to and parallel with the thenar crease and extends from just proximal to the wrist crease proximally, and as far as the level of the thumb web space, distally (Fig. 7.8). During incision, care is taken to preserve the small cutaneous nerves to avoid incisional tenderness. The TCL and related fascia are divided. The division is not complete until the median nerve can be seen throughout its course in the canal. Any adhesions of the median nerve to surrounding flexor tenosynovium are freed by careful dissection. The carpal tunnel floor is inspected for ganglia or bony spurs. The skin is closed with interrupted fine sutures.

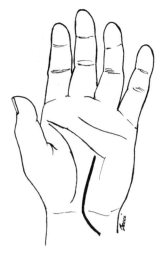

Figure 7.8. Skin incision for open carpal tunnel decompression.

2. Endoscopic carpal tunnel decompression

The past decade has seen the introduction of endoscopic carpal tunnel release as an alternative surgical procedure to open carpal tunnel release. The two best known techniques are the two-portal technique of Chow (1994) and the single portal technique of Agee et al. (1995).

The advantages of endoscopic release over open decompression include a faster return to activity and more rapid return of grip strength. The procedure does, however, carry a greater risk of iatrogenic injury because the median nerve is not actually seen during the procedure.

Pillar pain remains a problem that is associated with both the open and endoscopic techniques of decompression. Palm tenderness, usually associated with the open technique, has not been fully eliminated with endoscopic decompression.

Results

Relief of pain following surgery should be immediate; however, relief of numbness or weakness may be slow and incomplete. Nerve conductivity improves slowly over 1 to 2 years.

Complications of surgery

Intraoperative complications include injury to the median nerve trunk or its branches. Immediate postoperative complications include: haematoma (from damage to the superficial palmar arch), oedema or infection.

Later complications can include: persisting hand weakness, palmar pain/hypersensitivity from the entrapment of cutaneous nerves within the scar, pillar pain, hypertrophic scarring, palmar fasciitis and chronic regional pain syndrome resulting from injury to the palmar cutaneous branch of the nerve. This complication can lead to disability far greater than the original disorder.

Postoperative management

Exercise

The wound is dressed and supported with a light compression bandage. The hand is rested in neutral extension for the first 1 to 2 postoperative days. Neck, shoulder and elbow movements are commenced immediately to maintain longitudinal glide of the median nerve. Thumb and finger movements are performed within the postoperative cast.

Gentle active wrist movements are commenced on the 2nd or 3rd postoperative day. Specific median nerve gliding exercises are performed as for conservative management of CTS. All exercises are performed gently and slowly every 2 h within the limits of discomfort. Earlier concerns regarding the risk of tendon bowstringing with early mobilization have been dispelled (Nathan et al., 1993). Nonetheless, simultaneous wrist and finger flexion is avoided as this position makes the tendons most vulnerable to bowstringing.

Scar management

Sutures are usually removed about 10 days after surgery. Scar management is then commenced. Light massage, using oil or cream, is usually well tolerated and should be performed 4 to 6 times a day by the patient as part of a home programme.

Most postoperative scars resolve uneventfully within 4 to 6 weeks after surgery. Raised or persisting scar is managed with silicone gel. The area should be washed and dried thoroughly and be free of oily residue prior to application of the gel. The gel is held in place with Tubigrip stockinette of appropriate tension (Fig. 7.9).

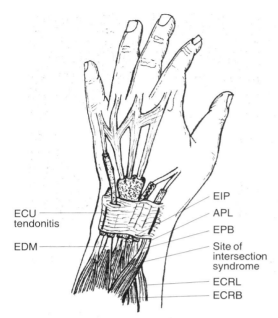

ECU tendonitis

EDM

EIP
APL
EPB
Site of intersection syndrome
ECRL
ECRB

Figure 8.1. The more common tendon disorders on the dorsum of the hand involve the 1st and 6th compartments, i.e. the tendons of abductor pollicis longus (APL)/extensor pollicis brevis (EPB) and extensor carpi ulnaris (ECU) respectively. Less common entrapment disorders involve the tendons of extensor indicis proprius (EIP) and extensor digiti minimi (EDM).

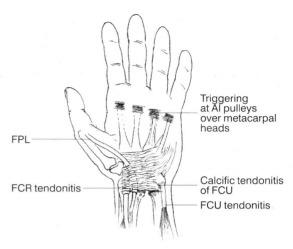

FPL

FCR tendonitis

Triggering at AI pulleys over metacarpal heads

Calcific tendonitis of FCU

FCU tendonitis

Figure 8.2. Common tendon disorders on the volar aspect of the hand include triggering of the thumb and/or digital flexor tendons and tendonitis of flexor carpi radialis (FCR) and flexor carpi ulnaris (FCU). The FCU tendon can be the site for calcific deposits near the tendon's junction with the pisiform. In rheumatoid disease, flexor pollicis longus (FPL) can undergo attrition rupture due to bony spicules on the scaphoid.

Patient presentation

The incidence of trigger finger peaks in the sixth decade of life. The thumb is most commonly affected, followed by the ring, middle, little and index fingers (Weilby, 1970). Several digits can be affected at once. Multiple digit involvement is more common in insulin-dependent diabetics who sometimes present with a mild PIP joint flexion deformity of the middle finger. Non-diabetic patients with longstanding triggering may also present with a PIP joint flexion deformity which is sometimes mistaken for Dupuytren's disease or joint dislocation.

The patient may complain of tenderness over the A1 pulley, pain on active flexion and/or 'catching' or 'clicking' of the PIP joint as the finger moves from extension to flexion or from flexion to full extension. The digit may actually 'lock' into flexion and require passive correction to restore digital extension. The thickened flexor sheath can generally be palpated.

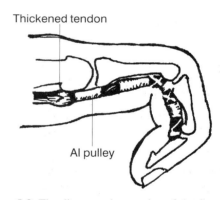

Thickened tendon

AI pulley

Figure 8.3. The disproportionate size of the flexor tendon in relation to its overlying retinacular pulley can result in pain on active flexion and cause the finger to 'trigger' or, in severe cases, lock into the flexed position.

Conservative management

1. Corticosteroid injection
Primary triggering of the digits can often be treated successfully with corticosteroid injection into the tendon sheath. Success of this treatment is greater in patients with involvement of only

one digit and where duration of symptoms is less than four months (Newport et al., 1990). If symptoms persist, the injection can be repeated on two more occasions without the risk of possible complications such as skin depigmentation, skin atrophy or tendon rupture (Marks and Gunther, 1989).

2. Splinting

Patients who do not wish to undergo injection or surgical release can be managed with a hand-based splint which immobilizes the MCP joint(s) of the affected digit(s) in neutral extension. This treatment protocol was devised by Evans et al. (1988) and its aim is to rest the proximal pulley system by altering the biomechanics of the flexor tendons (Fig. 8.4). The outcomes of splinting have been compared with those of injection at follow-up after one year and results have been encouraging. Sixty-six per cent of splinted digits were symptom-free compared to 84 per cent in the case of injected digits (Patel and Bassini, 1992).

The patient is asked to wear the splint during waking hours for an initial period of 3 weeks. The splint prevents flexion at the MCP joint(s) of affected digit(s), however is 'stepped down' to allow MCP flexion of uninvolved digits. Every 2 hours during the day, the patient actively flexes

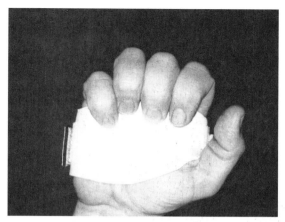

Figure 8.5. On a 2-hourly basis, the patient fully flexes and extends the digits 20 times. The purpose of this exercise is to maintain the differential glide of the flexor tendons.

the fingers into a 'hook fist' and then actively extends the digits to full range. This exercise maintains the differential glide of the flexor tendons within the sheath and is repeated 20 times at each session (Fig. 8.5).

At the completion of this set of exercises, 'place and hold' flexion exercises are performed in the full-fist position, i.e. the fingers are passively placed into full flexion at all three digital joints and the patient is then asked to gently maintain this fully flexed position for several seconds. This manoeuvre maintains mobility of the MCP joints and avoids the 'triggering' that can occur with active digital flexion from the fully extended position.

If the patient has shown some improvement during the 3-week period, a further 3 weeks of treatment can be trialled. If there has been no improvement during this time, steroid injection or pulley release are indicated.

Surgery

The pulley is generally divided through an open procedure; however, percutaneous trigger finger release is an alternative procedure (Stothard and Kumar, 1994). The percutaneous method is contra-indicated in patients with rheumatoid disease, diabetes or those with excessive subcutaneous tissue (Froimson, 1993) (Fig. 8.6).

Early active movement is begun within a day of surgery and scar management is commenced upon removal of sutures.

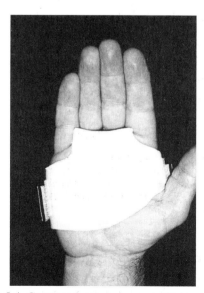

Figure 8.4. Conservative management of trigger finger(s) involves a hand-based splint that immobilizes the MCP joint(s) of the affected digit(s) in neutral extension.

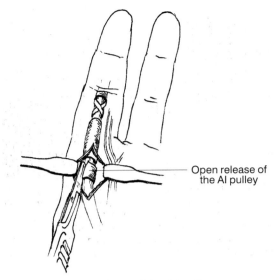

Figure 8.6. Open release of the A1 pulley.

2. de Quervain's disease

de Quervain's disease is stenosing tendovaginitis of the first dorsal compartment (Fig. 8.7). This is the most radial of the six dorsal extensor compartments and houses the sheaths of abductor pollicis longus (APL) and extensor pollicis brevis (EPB) at the radial styloid process. APL (which often has several slips) and EPB can share a tunnel or, more often, lie in separate tunnels. It has been suggested

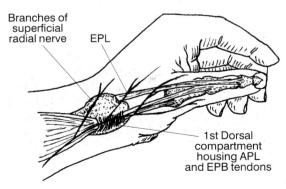

Figure 8.7. Stenosing tendovaginitis of the tendons in the first dorsal compartment (i.e. de Quervain's disease) involves the tendons of abductor pollicis longus (APL) and extensor pollicis brevis (EPB). Note the superficial branches of the radial nerve which are vulnerable to injury during decompression.

these anatomic anomalies may account for the poor response of some patients to conservative management (Minamikawa et al., 1991). There may be thickening of the retinacular roof, an associated ganglion and/or there may be radial nerve neuritis.

Aetiology

This condition can result from activities that require frequent thumb abduction in combination with ulnar deviation of the wrist. Occasionally, de Quervain's disease can present acutely from a local blunt injury to the styloid process.

Patient presentation

The patient generally presents with pain and swelling on the radial aspect of the wrist. The patient may complain of an ache in the thumb and this may radiate proximally into the forearm. Pain is aggravated by movement of the thumb. On palpation, there is tenderness over the radial styloid. If there is also involvement of the superficial branch of the radial nerve, sensitivity in this region can be quite marked.

Diagnostic manoeuvre

To help establish the diagnosis of de Quervain's disease, the following test is performed (Finkelstein, 1930). The patient is asked to flex the MCP and IP joints of the thumb across the palm. The fingers are then flexed over the thumb and the patient is asked to ulnar deviate the wrist. Where this manoeuvre elicits intense pain, the test is said to be positive. This manoeuvre can be uncomfortable in the normal wrist so comparison with the non-involved side should always be made (Fig. 8.8).

Resistance given to thumb extension at the level of the MCP joint can also be suggestive of EPB inflammation (Kirkpatrick and Lisser, 1995). This is referred to as the 'hitch-hiker's' test.

Differential diagnosis

Conditions that can present similarly to de Quervain's disease include arthritis of the first (CMC) joint (which may coexist with this condition) and, rarely, intersection syndrome where symptoms of pain and swelling of the APL and EPB muscle bellies occur 4–6 cm proximal to the

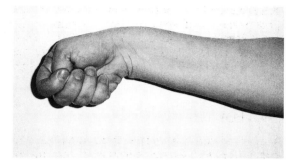

Figure 8.8. A positive Finkelstein test helps confirm the diagnosis for de Quervain's disease. This test involves flexing the thumb across the palm, then flexing the fingers over the thumb and ulnar deviating the wrist. While this manoeuvre is uncomfortable in the normal wrist, it usually elicits intense pain in patients with de Quervain's disease.

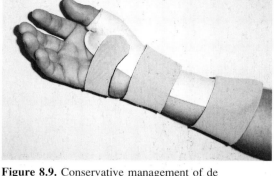

Figure 8.9. Conservative management of de Quervains's disease includes temporary immobilization in a thermoplastic splint that maintains the wrist in neutral or slight extension and the thumb in a functional degree of palmar abduction. The IP joint of the thumb is left free to move.

wrist rather than 1–2 cm as in the case of de Quervain's disease.

Conservative management

In the first instance, there should be cessation or modification of the precipitating activities. Splinting involves resting the wrist and thumb for a period of 3 to 4 weeks. The wrist is held in neutral or slight extension and the thumb is held in comfortable palmar abduction. The terminal joint of the thumb is left free to move (Fig. 8.9).

To expedite progress, splinting can be used in association with steroid injection into the synovial sheath of the first dorsal compartment. As in the case of triggering, conservative management of de Quervain's disease has a higher success rate in cases that are relatively acute. Success rate with steroid injection, given once or twice, ranges from 50 to 80 per cent (Harvey et al., 1990).

At the completion of the immobilization period, the patient can be fitted with a soft neoprene wrist/thumb wrap that provides elastic support without hindering movement. This support is particularly helpful for patients who are returning to work (Fig. 8.10).

Surgery

Surgical treatment involves decompression of the first dorsal compartment through either a transverse or longitudinal incision (Fig. 8.11). While a transverse incision leaves a more cosmetic scar,

exposure is compromised and the risk of injury to the superficial branch of the radial nerve is therefore greater. To avoid injury, the subcutaneous fat is incised by using gentle blunt longitudinal dissection. Under direct vision, the thickened compartment sheath is longitudinally incised on its dorsal surface. A volar lip of retinaculum is maintained to minimize the risk of volar dislocation of the APL tendon.

The compartment is explored for the presence of intervening septa which will require complete division. The tendons are decompressed from their musculotendinous junctions proximally, to about 1 cm distal to the retinaculum. The function of each tendon is tested for independent movement.

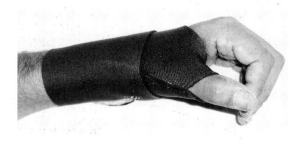

Figure 8.10. A soft neoprene thumb/wrist wrap provides support while allowing movement when activity is resumed.

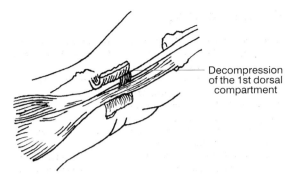

Decompression
of the 1st dorsal
compartment

Figure 8.11. The sheath of the 1st dorsal compartment is incised longitudinally on its dorsal surface. A volar lip of retinaculum is maintained to minimize the risk of volar dislocation of the APL tendon.

Aftercare

The wound is covered with a soft bulky dressing that restricts movement of the thumb for the first few postoperative days. Gentle active movement and light use of the hand is then begun.

Raised and/or sensitive scar is managed with Opsite Flexifix and silicone gel. Patients who develop problems of marked hypersensitivity from irritation of the radial nerve are also treated with transcutaneous electrical nerve stimulation.

3. Flexor carpi radialis

The tendon of flexor carpi radialis lies in its own tight fibrous canal and is anchored rigidly to the wall of the trapezium. This appears to render the tendon vulnerable to both primary tendovaginitis and to the secondary effects of carpal degeneration (Bishop et al., 1994).

Patient presentation

The patient is typically a middle-aged female who presents with pain over the scaphoid tubercle. There may be some local swelling and an overlying ganglion. When the patient is asked to actively flex and radially deviate the wrist against resistance, increased pain will help suggest the diagnosis (Fitton et al., 1968).

Treatment

This condition usually responds to a combination of rest in a wrist splint, non-steroidal anti-inflammatory medication and corticosteroid injection. Most cases settle within 2 to 3 weeks.

Where tendovaginitis is secondary to arthritic lesions, decompression of the tendon may be indicated to avoid attrition rupture.

4. Extensor carpi ulnaris

The tendon of extensor carpi ulnaris can become inflamed following a twisting injury of the wrist or repetitive hypersupination with wrist ulnar deviation. This condition, which presents with pain and swelling on the ulnar side of the wrist, can be difficult to distinguish from other pathology in this area, e.g. arthritis of the distal radioulnar joint or tears of the triangular fibrocartilage.

A provocative manoeuvre that points to the diagnosis involves giving resistance to wrist extension and ulnar deviation. This results in increased pain which may be accompanied by crepitus within the swollen sheath.

Treatment

Conservative treatment includes ice (in the immediate postinjury phase), wrist splinting in extension, anti-inflammatory medication and corticosteroid injection.

Where symptoms persist, decompression of the sixth dorsal compartment is carried out.

References

Bishop, A. T., Gabel, G. and Carmichael, S. W. (1994). Flexor carpi radialis tendinitis. Part 1: Operative anatomy. *J. Bone Joint Surg.,* **76A**, 1009–14.

Bunnell, S. (1944). Injuries of the hand. In *Surgery of the Hand.* pp. 496–9, Lippincott.

Evans, R. B., Hunter, J. M. and Burkhalter, W. E. (1988). Conservative management of the trigger finger: a new approach. *J. Hand Ther.,* **1**, 59.

Finkelstein, H. (1930). Stenosing tendovaginitis at the radial styloid process. *J. Bone Joint Surg.,* **12**, 509.

Fitton, J. M., Shea, W. F. and Goldie, W. (1968). Lesions of the flexor carpi radialis tendon and sheath causing pain at the wrist. *J. Bone Joint Surg.,* **50B**, 359–63.

Froimson, A. I. (1993). Tenosynovitis and tennis elbow. In *Green's Operative Hand Surgery* (D. P. Green, ed.), Churchill Livingstone.

Harvey, F. J., Harvey, P. M. and Horsley, M. W. (1990). De Quervain's disease: surgical or nonsurgical treatment. *J. Hand Surg.,* **15A**, 83–7.

Hueston, J. T., Wilson, W. F. and Soin, K. (1973). Trigger thumb. *Med. J. Aust.,* **2**, 1044–5.

Keon-Cohen, B. (1951). De Quervain's disease. *J. Bone Joint Surg.,* **33B**, 96–9.

Kirkpatrick, W. H. and Lisser, S. (1995). Soft tissue conditions: Trigger fingers and De Quervain's disease. In *Rehabilitation of the Hand: Surgery and Therapy* (J. M. Hunter, E. J. Mackin and A. D. Callahan, eds) pp. 1007–15.

Kozin, S. H. and Bishop, A. T. (1994). Atypical Mycobacterium infections of the upper extremity. *J. Hand Surg.,* **19A**, 480–7.

Marks, M. R. and Gunther, S. F. (1989). Efficacy of cortisone injection in treatment of trigger fingers and thumbs. *J. Hand Surg.,* **14A**, 722–7.

Minamikawa, Y., Peimer, C. A., Cox, W. L. and Sherwin, F. S. (1991). De Quervain's syndrome: surgical and anatomical studies of the fibro-osseous canal. *Orthopaedics,* **14**, 545–9.

Newport, M. L., Lane, L. B. and Stuchin, S. A. (1990). Treatment of trigger finger by steroid injection. *J. Hand Surg.,* **15A**, 748–50.

Patel, M. R. and Bassini, L. (1992). Trigger fingers and thumb: when to splint, inject or operate. *J. Hand Surg.,* **17A**, 110–3.

Stothard, J. and Kumar, A. (1994). A safe percutaneous procedure for trigger finger release. *J. R. Coll. Surg. Edinb.,* **39**, 116–7.

Weilby, A. (1970). Trigger finger. Incidence in children and adults and the possibility of a predisposition in certain age groups. *Acta Orthop. Scand.,* **41**, 419–27.

Wolfe, S. W. (1999). Tenosynovitis. In *Green's Operative Hand Surgery* (D. P. Green, R. N. Hotchkiss and W. C. Pederson, eds) pp. 2022–44, Churchill Livingstone.

Further reading

Arons, M. S. (1987). De Quervain's release in working women: a report of failures, complications and associated diagnoses. *J. Hand Surg.,* **12A**, 540–4.

Carroll, R. E., Sinton, W. and Garcia, A. (1955). Acute calcium deposits in the hand. *JAMA,* **157**, 422–6.

Phalen, G. S. (1991). Stenosing tenosynovitis: Trigger fingers, trigger thumb and De Quervain's disease. Acute calcification in wrist and hand. In *Flynn's Hand Surgery* (J. P. Jupiter, ed.) pp. 439–47, Williams & Wilkins.

Sampson, S. P., Badalamente, M. A., Hurst, L. C. and Seidman, J. (1991). Pathobiology of the human A1 pulley in trigger finger. *J. Hand Surg.,* **16A**, 714–21.

Sampson, S. P., Wisch, D. and Badalamente, M. A. (1994). Complications of conservative and surgical treatment of De Quervain's disease and trigger fingers. *Hand Clin.,* **10**, 73–82.

Secretan, H. (1901). Oedeme dur et hyperplasie traumatique du metacarpe dorsal. *Rev. Med. Suisse Romande.,* **21**, 409.

Shaw, J. A. (1986). Acute calcific tendonitis in the hand. *Orthop. Rev.,* **15**, 482–5.

Witt, J., Pess, G. and Gelberman, R. H. (1991). Treatment of De Quervain's tenosynovitis. A prospective study of the results of injection of steroids and immobilization in a splint. *J. Bone Joint Surg.,* **73A**, 219–22.

9

Dupuytren's contracture

Definition

Dupuytren's disease is a condition in which nodules and cords form in the palmar-digital fascia of the hand (Luck, 1959). The fascia undergoes pathological change which converts the normal bands and ligaments into diseased cords. These cords can displace neurovascular bundles and may cause soft tissue and joint contractures (Fig. 9.1). The pathologic tissue is comprised of immature collagen and fibroblasts.

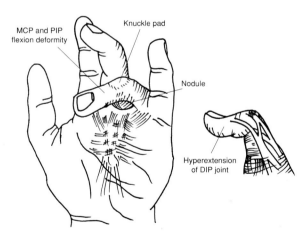

Figure 9.1. Features of the Dupuytren's hand can include: palmar cords and nodules, interdigital web contracture, flexion deformity at the MCP and/or PIP joints, hyperextension deformity of the DIP joint and knuckle pads. (Note the skip area where the skin is not tethered by the disease. Fat lying between the skin and the disease in this skip area will often contain the neurovascular bundle.)

Aetiology

The aetiology of this condition remains unknown. Current evidence points to a genetic predisposition. The disease is seen most frequently in the populations of northern Europe. It is rare amongst Oriental and black races.

The significance of injury or occupation as predisposing factors in the development of Dupuytren's disease remains controversial (Meagher, 1990). The disease is associated with certain medical conditions, e.g. diabetes and rheumatoid arthritis. Earlier associations with epilepsy point to the drugs used in treatment, rather than the condition itself, to account for the relationship (Hurst and Badalamente, 1990).

Patient presentation

The patient with Dupuytren's disease may present with a palmar or digital nodule, a cord or both (Fig. 9.2). The skin may or may not be involved. There may be contracture of a single digit involving one or all three joints or there may be involvement of multiple digits and one or more web spaces. Where the disease is present on the radial aspect of the hand, it is often more aggressive and difficult to treat. It is also usually more aggressive in the younger patient.

There may be extrapalmar ectopic deposits manifesting as knuckle pads, plantar nodules and Peyronie's disease. Unless associated with acute palmar fasciitis or carpal tunnel syndrome, Dupuytren's disease is usually painless.

The presenting hand may be supple and mobile or thick with joints that are prone to stiffness. The stiff,

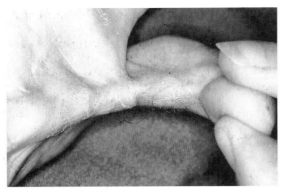

Figure 9.2. This little finger demonstrates a palmar nodule, a palmar-digital cord and a marked PIP joint flexion deformity. Note the skin excoriation.

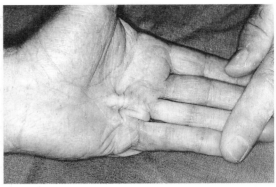

Figure 9.3. Contracture of the MCP joint is caused primarily by involvement of the pretendinous band.

arthritic or sweaty hand is prone to post-surgical complications. There can be associated triggering of the finger or carpal tunnel syndrome. These conditions are more likely in diabetic patients.

The average age of onset in men is about 48 years, while in women it is 59 years. Although the disease appears later in women, and is usually less severe, the postoperative complication of chronic regional pain syndrome is double that of men. The overall incidence of this complication is approximately 5 per cent.

Structures involved in contracture

MCP joint

Contracture of the metacarpophalangeal joint is caused primarily by involvement of the pretendinous band (Fig. 9.3). Contracture can also

result from diseased fascia of the intrinsic musculature. Disease of the natatory ligament causes web space contracture which will limit finger span.

PIP joint

The bands and ligaments which become diseased, resulting in contracture of the PIP joint, are several in number. Surgical correction of this joint is therefore more difficult. Of the various cords that can develop in the digit (i.e. lateral, central, natatory or spiral), it is contracture of the spiral cord that can significantly displace the neurovascular bundle, rendering it susceptible to injury during surgery (Umlas et al., 1994). The spiral cord is comprised of: the pretendinous band, the spiral band, the lateral digital sheet and Grayson's ligament (Fig. 9.4).

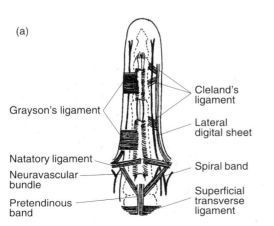

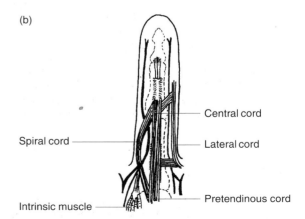

(a)

Grayson's ligament

Cleland's ligament

Lateral digital sheet

Natatory ligament

Neuravascular bundle

Pretendinous band

Spiral band

Superficial transverse ligament

(b)

Spiral cord

Intrinsic muscle

Central cord

Lateral cord

Pretendinous cord

Figure 9.4. (a) Normal components of the finger fascia. (b) When diseased, the normal components of the digital fascia are converted into the spiral, lateral and central cords which result in flexion contracture of the PIP joint.

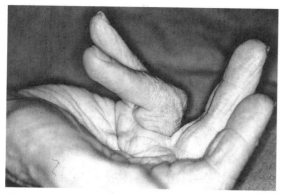

Figure 9.5. Surgery is indicated where the patient presents with a functional disability or where there has been rapid progression of the disease.

Indications for surgery

Surgery is indicated if the patient presents with a functional disability or where there has been rapid progression of the disease. Contractures of the PIP joint of 30 degrees or less are generally not treated by surgery (McFarlane and Botz, 1990). Such cases of mild deformity with slow progression are monitored on a 6 to 12 monthly basis (Fig. 9.5).

Limited surgery is advisable for the elderly patient. In the younger patient with a strong Dupuytren's diathesis and progressive contracture, more radical surgery is advised.

Patients who request surgical treatment for cosmetic reasons should be warned of the possible risk of losing some hand function. Most patients with Dupuytren's contracture can make a normal fist before surgery, but some may have difficulty regaining full flexion after surgery.

Biologically, the disease can extend beyond the field of surgical clearance. Cure of the disease by complete fasciectomy, therefore, is not possible. Because of the potential for a number of post-operative complications, e.g. ischaemia and infection, it is prudent to inform the patient of their possible occurrence.

Results

Approximately 80 per cent of patients can expect to gain a near-normal range of extension following surgery. Return of maximum flexion range can take some months, particularly in the older patient

with coexisting problems, e.g. osteoarthritis or diabetes.

Long-term results show a recurrence rate ranging from 25 to 80 per cent. Studies suggest that this rate is influenced not so much by the surgical technique as by the disease process itself. Full-thickness skin grafting alone has been shown by Hueston (1984a) to decrease recurrence rate.

Contraindications for surgery

These include the following:

1. Skin excoriation, maceration or infection, particularly in the web space.
2. Arthritis in the hand which is likely to be exacerbated by surgery.
3. A patient who is unable to comply with the postoperative therapy regimen.
4. Poor general health.

Types of incision

Palmar-digital contractures are approached through a longitudinal incision which is converted to a Z-plasty at closure. Transverse disease in the palm can be approached by a mid-palmar incision. A combined thumb and thumb web contracture is approached by an incision both along the thumb ray and the thumb web. Both incisions are converted to a single or double Z-plasty at closure (Fig. 9.6).

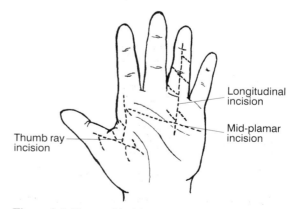

Figure 9.6. Types of incision.

to wound and other hand complications (... and Conolly, 1996):

function.

10

Fractures of the hand

Jacki Shannon-Johnstone

Fractures to the hand are common and most can be treated conservatively by simple closed reduction, protective splinting and early mobilization (Pun et al., 1989). Non-operative treatment is preferred wherever possible to avoid further trauma to the soft tissues, thus ensuring a more favourable outcome.

The most commonly fractured bone in the hand is the distal phalanx, accounting for nearly 50 per cent of all hand fractures. Metacarpal fractures account for approximately 30 per cent of fractures. The remaining 20 per cent occur in the proximal and middle phalanges (Meyer and Wilson, 1995).

Assessment

1. Mechanism of injury

The mechanism of injury will determine the type of fracture. A direct blow will usually result in a transverse fracture. These tend to produce angulatory deformities which can be seen in both lateral and frontal radiographic views. A spiral or oblique fracture results from a twisting injury. Oblique fractures result in rotatory deformities but may also angulate or shorten. Crushing injuries produce comminuted fractures which nearly always shorten and may rotate or angulate. The degree of soft tissue injury associated with the fracture has a direct correlation to the final range of motion (Duncan et al., 1993).

Rotational deformity can be assessed by noting the position of the fingernails when the digits are extended. They generally lie in the same plane as one another. Orientation of the fingers should be compared with the opposite hand. During flexion, fingers are checked for a tendency to cross over one another, i.e. 'scissor'.

2. Radiological examination

Good quality X-rays are essential for accurate diagnosis. Three views are required: anteroposterior (AP), oblique and lateral. Oblique views are particularly important for the assessment of intra-articular fractures.

3. Soft tissue injury

Because stress testing for ligament damage has the potential to displace a fracture, it should be carried out after fracture evaluation. Local anaesthetic should be administered prior to the test to eliminate pain.

Classification of fractures

Fractures of the metacarpals and phalanges can be classified in the following way (Fig. 10.1):

1. Closed or open.
2. Stable or unstable.
3. According to fracture geometry, i.e. transverse, oblique, spiral or comminuted.
4. According to site, i.e. base, shaft, neck or head.
5. According to fracture deformity, i.e. rotational, angular or shortening.

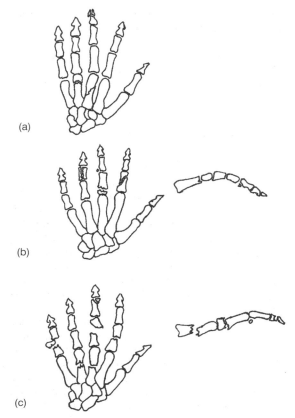

(a)

(b)

(c)

Figure 10.1. Classification of fractures. (a) Stable; (b) potentially unstable; (c) unstable.

6. Intra-articular or extra-articular.
7. By the presence or absence of associated ligament, tendon or neurovascular injuries.

Stable fractures

A fracture is considered stable if the bone fragments do not displace when stress is applied. Stable fractures may require temporary splinting to support the soft tissue and to relieve pain. Gentle active range of movement can usually be commenced several days following injury.

Displaced metacarpal and phalangeal fractures can often undergo closed reduction. Appropriate analgesia will be required and an X-ray should be taken prior to and post reduction to ensure bony alignment has been achieved.

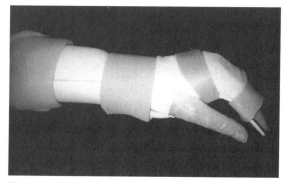

Figure 10.2. The hand is placed in the 'position of safe immobilization' following fracture reduction.

Position of safe immobilization

Following reduction the hand is rested in the position of safe immobilization, i.e. in a POSI splint (Fig. 10.2). This position is also referred to as the 'intrinsic plus' or 'clam-digger' position and is as follows:

1. Wrist extension of 30 to 40 degrees.
2. Maximum MCP joint flexion (usually 80 to 90 degrees).
3. Maximum interphalangeal joint extension (ideally 0 degrees).

The position of safe immobilization maintains the collateral ligaments of all finger joints at optimal length thereby avoiding the tendency toward extension contracture of the MCP joints and flexion contracture of the PIP joints. Both these contractures are commonly associated with fractures of the hand (Fig. 10.3).

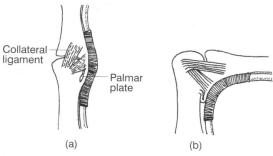

Figure 10.3. The collateral ligaments of the MCP joints are (a) relaxed and short when the joints are extended and (b) stretched when the joints are flexed.

Unstable fractures

In an unstable fracture, bony alignment is easily lost. Internal fixation is needed to restore and maintain normal bony anatomy.

Open reduction and internal fixation

Approximately 10 per cent of phalangeal and metacarpal fractures require open reduction and internal fixation (Melone, 1986). Open reduction has gained greater acceptance over the past two decades due to increased understanding of the biomechanical principles of internal fixation, improved materials, increasing specialization in surgery of the hand and antibiotic availability to minimize the risk of infection.

Indications for open reduction and internal fixation are:

1. Unstable fracture where closed reduction cannot be achieved or maintained.
2. Intra-articular fractures.
3. Multiple fractures.
4. Open fractures, particularly where there is bone loss.
5. Fractures associated with soft tissue damage requiring surgery, e.g. tendon and/or nerve damage.
6. Rotational malalignment, usually seen in spiral and oblique fractures.
7. Pathological fractures (e.g. enchondroma).
8. Malunion or non-union.
9. Reconstruction, e.g. rotation osteotomy for malunion.

The advantages of open reduction and internal fixation of hand fractures are:

1. Screws and plates provide more stability.
2. The reduction is more accurate.
3. Movement can be commenced within a day or two of surgery.

Fixation methods (Fig. 10.4)

1. Kirschner wires

Kirschner wires (K-wires) offer the simplest technique for fracture fixation and because they can be inserted percutaneously, they can be placed with minimal soft tissue dissection. They can be used for nearly all types of fracture. Crossed K-wires are most suited for transverse fractures. In long oblique fractures the wire is placed perpendicular to the bone. In spiral fractures they are placed in parallel. Some surgeons prefer to bury the pin while others prefer to let it protrude through the skin.

While a simple and relatively cheap technique, K-wires often require support splinting or supplementary techniques as they do not provide rigid internal fixation. They are unsuitable for comminuted or open fractures or in association with significant soft tissue injury. The complication rate associated with the use of K-wires in the hand and wrist is 18 per cent (Botte et al., 1992).

2. Wiring

Because K-wires on their own do not provide rigid fixation or rotational stability, they are often

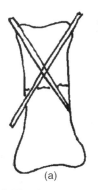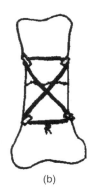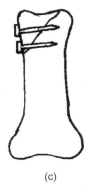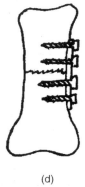

Figure 10.4. Fixation methods. (a) Crossed Kirschner wires are most suited for transverse fractures; (b) composite wiring converts distraction forces into compression forces; (c) lag (or compression) screws can provide rigid fixation; (d) plating provides longitudinal stability that can resist bending as well as torsional forces.

supplemented by wiring (composite wiring). This combined technique allows early active movement.

Composite wiring converts distraction forces into compression forces at the fracture site and is particularly suitable for unstable transverse or short oblique phalangeal fractures. The interosseous tension band wire is passed as a figure of eight, with the crossover lying external to the two fracture fragments.

Interosseous wiring requires minimal exposure and is less prominent than plates or screws. It is useful for transverse shaft fractures. Because this form of fixation does not interfere with mobility of adjacent joints, it is particularly suited to replantation and fusion.

3. Lag (or compression) screw

The lag or compression screw allows two fragments to be compressed together. Compression of the fracture surfaces gives rigid fixation. This form of fixation is best suited to long oblique and spiral shaft fractures when the fracture length is at least twice the diameter of the bone. Maximum compression is achieved with the screw at right angles to the fracture plane. A single lag screw is ideal for a small fracture fragment such as a unicondylar fracture of the head of the proximal phalanx.

4. Plates

Plating provides longitudinal stability that can resist bending as well as torsional forces. Plating is particularly suitable for multiple fractures, especially those associated with soft tissue injury or for bone loss requiring grafting (Simonetta, 1970). They are also appropriate for unstable transverse fractures in a single digit. Compression screws may be inserted through the plate's holes if they are at suitable angles or they may be inserted away from the plate. Micro-plates from maxillofacial sets (Luhr Microfixation system) are now being utilized. These plates are low profile, thus allowing the periosteum to be closed with less tendency toward adhesion formation.

5. Intramedullary fixation

Open reduction and intramedullary fixation can be achieved in transverse metacarpal shaft fractures using a Steinmann pin. Early active movement can be commenced with this form of fixation. This technique is not suitable for long oblique or spiral metacarpal fractures.

A closed technique of intramedullary fixation is now available. This technique involves the use of three blunt and pre-bent flexible K-wires that ensure rotational control through 3-point fixation. This technique has been described by Foucher (1995) in the management of displaced fractures of the fifth metacarpal neck and is known as 'bouquet osteosynthesis'.

6. External fixation

External fixation is reserved for severe fractures where restoration of the skeletal anatomy is not possible. These include comminuted open fractures which are often associated with bone loss and/or damage to soft tissues, i.e. tendon and nerve. External fixators can function either statically or dynamically.

(i) Static fixator
A static fixator can be used across the MCP joint of the thumb for a comminuted intra-articular fracture. Stiffness at this joint can be compensated for by the mobility of the basal thumb joint, i.e. the CMC joint.

(ii) Dynamic fixator
Dynamic traction combines the old method of traction with motion and can be used for unstable intra-articular PIP joint fractures, e.g. pilon fractures. The two types of dynamic traction include the arcuate splint and the low profile lateral hinge traction splint (Dennys et al., 1992). The distal distraction produces several effects. The articular fragments are reduced and the joint surfaces realigned by traction on their ligamentous and volar plate attachments. This process is termed ligamentotaxis. Maintenance of traction throughout the healing process prevents collapse of the fracture fragments. Furthermore, the distal distraction force prevents contracture of the joint ligaments and other periarticular structures. Joint motion enhances cartilage regeneration and healing (see 'Joint injuries of the fingers and thumb').

Complications associated with fractures

1. Delayed union or non-union caused by infection, poor blood supply, interspersed fragments of tissue such as muscle, or movement of the fractured parts.
2. Malunion, rotation of a spiral fracture or angulation of a transverse fracture.

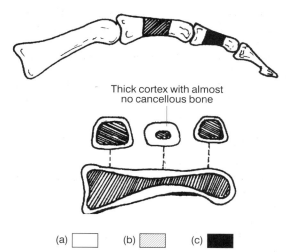

Thick cortex with almost no cancellous bone

(a) ☐   (b) ▨   (c) ■

Figure 10.5. Healing timetable for bone. Fracture consolidation varies within each segment of the hand and is slowest where the ratio of cortical to cancellous bone is highest. (a) 3–5 weeks; (b) 5–7 weeks; (c) 10–14 weeks. (From Moberg, 1950, with permission).

3. Adherence of the closely allied flexor/extensor tendons resulting from postinjury oedema and/or surgery.
4. Joint stiffness and contracture, i.e. extension contracture of the MCP joints after metacarpal fractures or flexion contracture of the PIP joint following phalangeal fracture.
5. Occasionally, development of chronic regional pain syndrome.

Phases of bone healing (Fig. 10.5)

Following a fracture, bone healing occurs in three overlapping phases:

1. Inflammatory phase

This phase occurs in the 3 to 4 days following a fracture. The gap in the bone is bridged with a blood clot which coagulates to form a haematoma. An inflammatory response is triggered by mediators released from dead and injured cells. This results in vasodilation, plasma exudation and migration of inflammatory cells to the fracture site. Osteoclasts resorb dead bone and fibroblasts start producing a new matrix (Fig. 10.6(a)).

2. Reparative phase

The fracture haematoma begins to organize. Fibrin in the haematoma provides a framework for

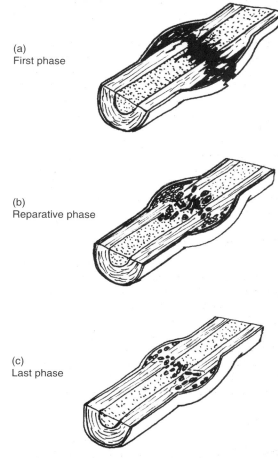

(a)
First phase

(b)
Reparative phase

(c)
Last phase

Figure 10.6. Diagrammatic representation of the three phases of fracture healing. (Reproduced from Meyer, F. N. and Wilson, R. L. 1995. Management of nonarticular fractures of the hand. In *Rehabilitation of the Hand: Surgery and Therapy* (J. M. Hunter, E. J. Mackin and A. D. Callahan, eds) p. 354, Mosby, with permission.)

migration of fibroblasts and undifferentiated mesenchymal cells. There is ingrowth of capillary buds. The cells increase in number and differentiate into what is known as fracture callus. The centre of the inflammatory reaction is made up of mostly cartilage, called soft callus. This soft callus is gradually replaced by bone. The immature bone being formed at the periphery of this reaction is called hard callus.

By the end of this phase, which usually lasts 4 to 6 weeks, a fracture may be considered clinically healed, i.e. there is no motion at the fracture site when stressed and no pain with active movement of nearby joints. At this stage there is usually little radiographic evidence of fracture healing. Clinical healing occurs in about a quarter of the time it takes for complete bony healing to occur (Smith and Rider, 1935) (Fig. 10.6(b)).

3. Remodelling phase

During this phase lamellar bone replaces woven bone and callus is resorbed. Much of this phase occurs in the first few months after injury; however, this phase can continue for several years (Fig. 10.6(c)).

Primary bone healing

When the fractured bone ends are brought into direct contact with one another, i.e. with open reduction and internal fixation, primary bone healing occurs in two phases: gap healing and haversian remodelling.

Lamellar bone forms directly across the fracture site. Osteoclasts bridge the fracture line followed by osteoblasts, which form new bone. Osteoblasts are followed by new capillaries. This forms new haversian systems called primary osteons.

Metacarpal fractures

1. Shaft fractures

(i) Transverse (Fig. 10.7)

In a transverse fracture, the interosseous muscles are responsible for dorsal angulation at the fracture site. Where angulation results in shortening of the metacarpal, compensatory hyperextension of the MCP joint will be present, i.e. a pseudo-claw. Mild angulation in the ring and little fingers is considered acceptable (20 and 30 degrees, respectively) because of compensatory mobility of the CMC joints in these two digits. Angulation of the less mobile index and middle fingers, however, is an indication for reduction and percutaneous pinning.

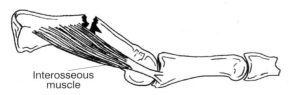

Figure 10.7. In a transverse metacarpal fracture, the interosseous muscles are responsible for dorsal angulation at the fracture site.

Interosseous muscle

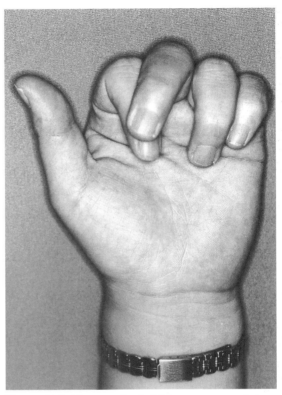

Figure 10.8. Metacarpal spiral fractures can result in rotational malalignment causing 'scissoring' of the digits during flexion.

(ii) Oblique and spiral

Oblique metacarpal fractures have a tendency to shorten. Where this exceeds 3–5 mm, an imbalance between the extrinsic and intrinsic muscles can result. Spiral fractures can result in rotational malalignment. Even a minor rotational deformity can be quite disabling as it will result in 'scissoring' of the digits during finger flexion (Opgrande and Westphal, 1983). This problem is best managed with open reduction (Fig. 10.8).

Conservative treatment and therapy

Splint position and oedema control

Most shaft fractures can be successfully managed closed. After fracture reduction, the hand is maintained for 3 to 4 weeks in the position of safe immobilization, i.e. wrist in 30 to 40 degrees of extension, MCP joints in maximum flexion and IP joints in maximum extension. A half-plaster applied

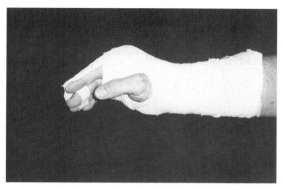

Figure 10.9. The hand is placed in the 'clam-digger' position (also known as the 'intrinsic plus' position or 'position of safe immobilization') with a dorsal half-plaster which will allow finger flexion and intrinsic IP joint extension to the limit of the splint.

to the dorsum of the forearm and hand will apply gentle compression to hand oedema and will allow unimpeded finger flexion and intrinsic IP joint extension to the limit of the cast (Fig. 10.9).

Because dorsal hand oedema is often marked, it may be difficult to place the MCP joints in maximum flexion (usually 80–90 degrees) at the initial cast application. The cast will therefore need to be replaced after several days when swelling has subsided. Coban wrap (50 mm width) or tubular support stocking (of appropriate tension) can be applied to the hand prior to moulding to assist with oedema resolution. The hand should be kept elevated for at least the 1st week.

Finger alignment

Alignment of the fingernails is assessed to check any tendency toward rotation of the affected digit. During interphalangeal flexion, the digit is observed for any tendency to cross over an adjacent digit. If the fracture has not been satisfactorily reduced, open reduction may be necessary.

Exercises

The patient should perform active shoulder and elbow exercises on an hourly basis during the 3 to 4 week splinting period. These proximal joint exercises are followed by gentle active combined (i.e. simultaneous PIP and DIP joint) interphalangeal joint flexion. Intrinsic extension of the IP joints should follow each flexion exercise and the patient should aim to reach the level of the

splint, i.e. full IP joint extension. These exercises are repeated 6 to 10 times at each session. To help maintain digital alignment, the affected digit can be buddy-strapped to an adjacent digit during active exercise.

At the completion of the splinting period, a lycra compression glove is fitted if dorsal hand oedema persists. The patient is taught to initiate fist-making at the MCP joints otherwise the natural tendency, in the presence of persisting oedema, will be to assume a hook grip where flexion is initiated at the IP joints whilst the MCP joints remain in extension. Light activity is commenced following plaster removal. Heavy use of the hand is avoided until 12 weeks post fracture.

Therapy following open reduction and internal fixation (ORIF)

Therapy following ORIF is much the same as for conservative management (Fig. 10.10). The main difference is that the postoperative splint can be removed for exercise sessions every few hours and can be discarded after 10 to 14 days when sutures are removed.

Oedema

Postoperative oedema is often marked, making flexion of the MCP joints difficult. Oedema should be managed with Coban wrap initially. Following suture removal, a lycra glove is fitted. If gentle passive/active exercise does not overcome MCP joint stiffness within the first 2 weeks, a dynamic MCP joint flexion splint should be applied (Fig. 10.11).

Extensor lag

Extensor tendon adhesion following surgery is quite common and can result in a temporary lag until tethering of the tendon to skin and bone is overcome. Scar massage, silicone gel compression and extrinsic extension exercises should be employed to address this problem.

Corrective procedures
(i) Wedge osteotomy

Dorsal angulation following transverse shaft fractures can result in prominence of the metacarpal head in the palm that causes pain when gripping. This deformity is also associated with a pseudo-claw due to shortening of the metacarpal. This

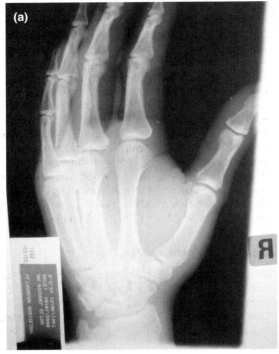

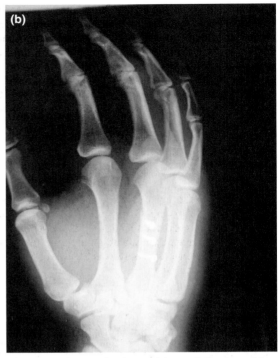

Figure 10.10. (a) Oblique fracture of the middle finger metacarpal; (b) Open reduction and internal fixation with compression screws.

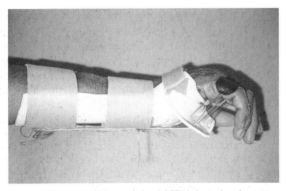

Figure 10.11. Stiffness of the MCP joints that is not readily overcome with passive/active exercise, is managed with a dynamic flexion splint.

problem can be addressed with an opening or closing wedge osteotomy.

(ii) Rotation osteotomy

Rotational malunion following spiral or oblique fractures can be addressed with a corrective osteotomy through the base of the metacarpal.

2. Neck fractures

Metacarpal neck fractures usually involve the ring and little finger metacarpals and result from the forceful impact of the clenched fist with a solid object.

There is not universal agreement on the management of these fractures. Treatment strategies vary considerably from centre to centre and include:

(i)   Crepe bandage support with immediate commencement of active movement.
(ii) Closed reduction and transverse percutaneous K-wire fixation of the fractured metacarpal to the adjacent metacarpal. Support splinting in the position of safe immobilization is used for 3 to 4 weeks, however the splint is removed every 2 to 3 hours during the day and gentle active exercise of all digits is carried out.
(iii) 'Bouquet osteosynthesis', i.e. closed intramedullary fixation using three pre-bent flexible K-wires (Foucher, 1995).
(iv) Open reduction, e.g. lateral application of a minicondylar plate.

Whatever treatment method is used, non-union is rarely a problem. Some patients are unhappy over the loss of prominence of the metacarpal head although this is more a cosmetic rather than a functional consideration.

Some surgeons believe that in the case of the little finger, significant angulation (up to 70 degrees) can be accepted without compromising function (Holst-Nielsen, 1976).

Metacarpal head and base fractures

1. Head

A fracture to the head of a metacarpal is rare and usually intra-articular. Comminuted intra-articular fractures can be difficult to treat with ORIF and in some cases immediate arthroplasty may be considered. An alternative option is an osteochondral autograft taken from a toe.

2. Base

Base fractures of the index and middle finger metacarpals are rare. Fracture dislocation of the little finger CMC joint is more common. Treatment options include closed reduction with percutaneous K-wire fixation or open reduction and internal fixation.

Fractures of the proximal and middle phalanges

1. Stable – conservative treatment

Fractures that are stable, closed and non-displaced are treated with a finger splint holding the interphalangeal joints in extension for 3 weeks. The splint is removed every few hours for gentle active IP joint flexion and extension exercises. Digital oedema is managed with a single layer of Coban wrap (25 mm) which is applied in a distal to proximal direction. A buddy strap can be used during active movement. A short section of narrow Coban can be used for this purpose (Fig. 10.12).

(i) Transverse fractures

Displaced fractures that are stable following reduction are splinted in the position of safe immobilization for 3 weeks. Transverse fractures of the proximal and middle phalanx are particularly amenable to closed reduction. Full extension of the interphalangeal joints may not be achievable when

the splint is first fitted. It should therefore be remoulded or replaced 3 to 5 days later. When the immediate soft tissue response of pain and swelling has subsided after the first 2 to 3 days, gentle active interphalangeal joint movement is begun.

To help control fracture alignment, the digit is buddy-strapped to an adjacent digit with nonstick strapping such as Velcro or a section of Coban. The splint is removed every 2 to 3 hours during the day and 5 to 10 repetitions of combined IP joint flexion and extension movements are performed. These exercises are carried out slowly within the limits of discomfort. Blocking the MCP joints in extension will help facilitate extrinsic flexor tendon pull-through. Following splint removal, buddy-strapping is maintained for a further 2 weeks.

(ii) Spiral fractures (Fig. 10.17)

Closed reduction of spiral fractures of the proximal and middle phalanges is often lost through early movement. For this reason, these fractures are immobilized in a POSI splint for 3 weeks (See Figure 10.2). Gentle active movement is then begun.

Associated problems

Flexion deformity of the PIP joint

As with any injury to the digits, the commonest complication after phalangeal fracture is a PIP joint flexion deformity. Coban wrap, with its gentle extension force, goes some way toward counteracting this problem. Maintenance of the digit in extension during splinting also helps avoid a flexion deformity. When the support splint is discarded after the 3rd week, a neoprene fingerstall will effectively maintain extension while at the same time allowing IP joint flexion (Fig. 10.13). A Capener splint is used if the flexion deformity is unresponsive to the neoprene stall.

Stiffness

If interphalangeal joint flexion range is slow to improve or has plateaued, flexion splinting can be instituted when clinical union has been achieved, usually 3 to 5 weeks following fracture (Fig. 10.14). Confirmation of skeletal integrity by the treating surgeon should be sought prior to the commencement of flexion splinting. This can involve gentle flexion bandaging, a hand-based dynamic flexion splint or an IP joint flexion strap to gain the end

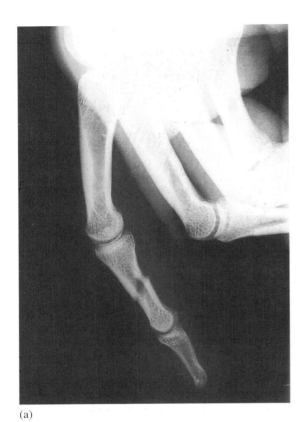

(a)

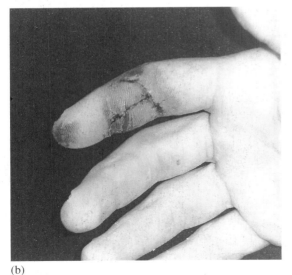

(b)

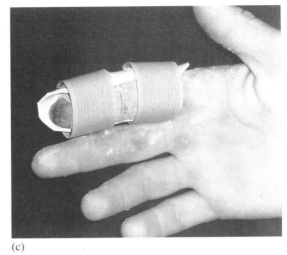

(c)

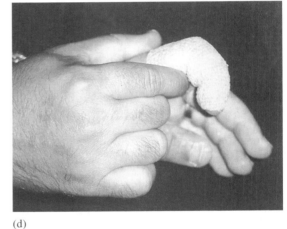

(d)

Figure 10.12. (a) This midshaft fracture of the middle phalanx of the middle finger is stable, non-displaced and was treated conservatively. (b) This fracture was associated with soft tissue injury. (c) Stable proximal and middle phalangeal fractures are protected with a finger splint for 3 weeks. Digital oedema is treated with Coban wrap (25 mm). (d) Gentle active interphalangeal joint flexion and extension exercises are performed every few hours.

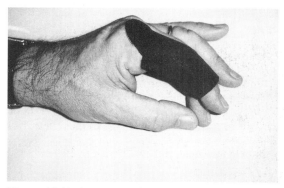

Figure 10.13. A neoprene fingerstall is an effective measure for controlling and overcoming flexion deformity of the PIP joint.

range of flexion (Fig. 10.15). Whatever method is used, care must be taken to apply only a gentle stretch which does not result in pain or swelling.

Functional outcome

The final range of motion achieved will be determined by a number of factors. These include:

1. Age of the patient.
2. The nature of the fracture and associated soft tissue injury, i.e. tendon, nerve and vessel injury or skin loss.
3. Length of immobilization.
4. Patient compliance and associated conditions, e.g. arthritis.

Of these various factors, the most significant one is the age of the patient. Patients in the first two decades of life achieve significantly greater mobility than those beyond the fourth or fifth decades. The patient with an underlying arthritic condition will be considerably more prone to stiffness. Excessive immobilization following fracture, i.e. beyond 4 weeks, is also responsible for a poor outcome (Strickland et al., 1982).

2. Unstable

(i) Closed reduction and percutaneous K-wire fixation

Shaft fractures that are potentially unstable can be addressed with percutaneous K-wire fixation for 3 weeks (Belsky and Eaton, 1985). These include

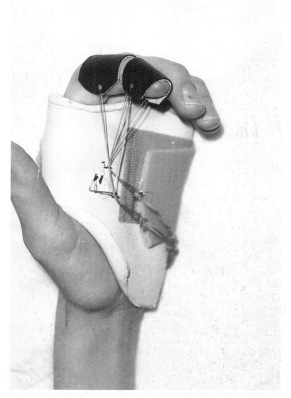

Figure 10.14. Stiffness of the PIP/DIP joint(s) is addressed with a hand-based dynamic flexion splint.

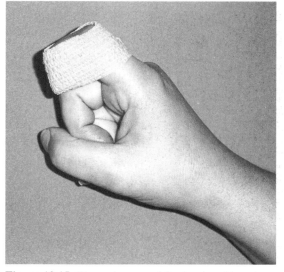

Figure 10.15. The end range of flexion is achieved with an IP joint flexion strap. Coban wrap (25 mm) was used in this instance.

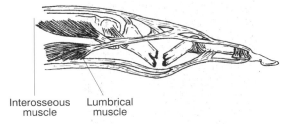

Interosseous   Lumbrical
muscle   muscle

Figure 10.16. The lumbricals and interossei are the deforming forces in a transverse proximal phalangeal fracture.

spiral and oblique fractures that tend to rotate, angulate or shorten. Most fractures needing percutaneous pinning will require two pins for stability and to control rotation.

This form of fixation is augmented with a support splint holding the hand in the position of safe immobilization. Ideally the fixation will be stable enough to allow early active movement several days after surgery. The splint is worn between exercise periods.

(ii) Rigid internal fixation

Irreducible spiral, oblique or transverse shaft fractures of the proximal and middle phalanges are best treated with rigid internal fixation. The potential problem of postoperative scarring following extensive soft tissue dissection is offset by the commencement of early active movement. Use of the lower profile Luhr microfixation system has allowed easier wound closure and less interference with extensor tendon excursion (Fig. 10.18).

Therapy

(a) Splinting and early movement

The hand is rested in a POSI splint for the first 3 to 5 postoperative days. Elevation is maintained and movement of the shoulder and elbow joints encouraged. If pain and swelling allow, the forearm-based splint can be replaced with a finger splint after about 5 days.

Gentle, active stabilized movement of the interphalangeal joints is begun 2 to 3 days following

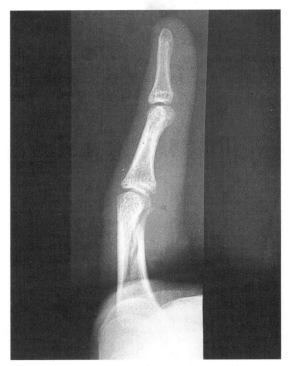

Figure 10.17. This potentially unstable proximal phalangeal fracture was treated conservatively with splinting in the 'position of safe immobilization'.

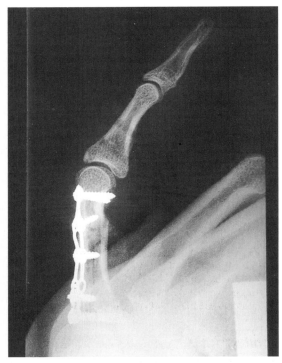

Figure 10.18. Irreducible fractures are treated with rigid internal fixation. The Luhr microfixation system was used to manage this unstable proximal phalangeal fracture.

surgery. Coban wrap (25 mm) can be applied over the dressing to reduce oedema. The finger splint is moulded over the Coban which is liberally coated with powder to prevent the heated material from sticking to the wrap. If maximum extension of the IP joints cannot be achieved at the initial splinting session, the finger splint should be replaced or remoulded several days later when swelling has further subsided. Support splinting is maintained for 3 to 5 weeks.

(b) Scar management

Following suture removal, soft tissue scarring is addressed with oil massage. Scar compression is also provided by Coban wrap, a neoprene finger-stall or silicone-lined fingerstalls. All these materials allow interphalangeal joint flexion.

(c) Stiffness

Stiffness of the PIP and DIP joints can be addressed with gentle flexion bandaging after the first two weeks. The tension of the bandage should be low and not result in pain. The effectiveness of flexion bandaging is augmented by immersing the hand in warm water for the 15 min that this position is maintained. This manoeuvre is repeated every few hours throughout the day. Where necessary, a hand-based dynamic flexion splint can be applied with the permission of the treating surgeon.

Fractures of the distal phalanx

The thumb and middle finger distal phalanges are the most common fracture sites in the hand. Most of these fractures are sustained in the workplace. Fractures of the distal phalanx can occur at three levels:

1. Tuft

These fractures invariably result from a crush injury and are often associated with laceration to the pulp and/or nail matrix. Closed injuries often result in a subungual haematoma which should be decompressed to provide relief of pain (Fig. 10.19).

Treatment

Treatment of these fractures involves repair of the nail matrix together with a short period of DIP joint support (7 to 10 days) to provide symptomatic relief. Dressings should be nonstick, e.g. Adaptic,

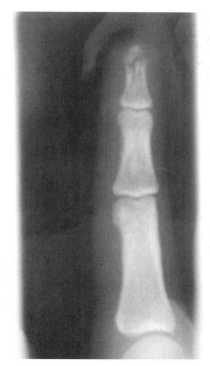

Figure 10.19. The distal phalanges of the thumb and middle finger are the most common fracture sites in the hand.

and can be held in place with gentle Coban compression. Movement of the more proximal joints is commenced immediately. On healing of the pulp, desensitization exercises are begun. To help alleviate hypersensitivity, Opsite Flexifix is applied over the sensitive area.

2. Shaft

Shaft fractures are either transverse or longitudinal. Unless displaced, these fractures can be treated conservatively for 2 to 3 weeks with a small thermoplastic splint which allows motion of the PIP joint.

Displaced fractures are stabilized with a Herbert screw or K-wire.

3. Base

Fractures to the base of the distal phalanx are often unstable and may require fixation, particularly if the injury is an open one. A stable fracture can be splinted in a mallet-type splint for 3 to 4 weeks.

Fractures of the distal phalanx are frequently associated with some long-term problems which include: numbness, cold sensitivity, hypersensitivity and abnormal nail growth.

Fractures to the thumb

Thumb fractures tend to be much more forgiving than finger fractures because of the compensatory movements afforded by the mobility of the thumb at its basal joint. The surfaces of the trapezium and thumb metacarpal resemble two interlocking saddles. This configuration allows motion in two planes. When the integrity of this joint is lost through injury or degenerative arthritis, thumb function is compromised. The thumb metacarpal is the second most commonly fractured metacarpal with 80 per cent of fractures occurring at its base.

1. Bennett's fracture

This intra-articular fracture was first described in 1882 by E. H. Bennett and is really a fracture subluxation. It usually involves less than a third of the articular surface. The fracture occurs at the medial volar lip which remains attached to the metacarpotrapezial ligament while the metacarpal shaft is subluxed radially and dorsally by the tendon of abductor pollicis longus. A true lateral view of the CMC joint must be obtained to establish joint congruity (Billing and Gedda, 1952).

(i). Closed reduction

In general, closed reduction alone is difficult because the pull of abductor pollicis longus tends to cause the base of the metacarpal to slide down the inclined plane of the trapezium.

In a low demand patient, particularly if the fragment is less than 15 to 20 per cent of the articular surface, percutaneous K-wire fixation and plaster immobilization for one month may be indicated. Pin fixation can be intermetacarpal, i.e. inserted between the thumb and index metacarpals, or through the metacarpal shaft and into the fractured fragment.

Aftercare

The thumb is immobilized in a forearm-based thumb spica for one month. A temporary plaster is fitted for the first few days after which the plaster is remade or a thermoplastic splint fitted to accommodate reduction of oedema. The thumb IP joint should be left free to move.

Following K-wire removal after 4 weeks, a removable splint is used for a further month of protection in between exercise sessions.

(ii) Open reduction and internal fixation

Where the patient has greater demand placed on the hand, e.g. a professional athlete, or where the fragment is greater than 25 to 30 per cent of the articular surface, open reduction and internal fixation with lag screws is preferred.

Aftercare

The thumb is protected in a forearm-based thumb spica for the first 10 to 14 days following surgery. The splint should maintain the first web space and the thumb should be aligned with the index and middle fingers. The splint is worn in 'at risk' situations for a further 2 to 3 weeks.

Gentle active movement of all thumb joints is begun 2 to 3 days after surgery. Contact sports can usually be resumed after 1 month.

2. Rolando's fracture (Fig. 10.20)

The Rolando fracture is also an intra-articular fracture and appears Y- or T-shaped. Anatomic

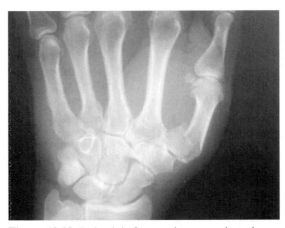

Figure 10.20. Rolando's fracture is a comminuted intra-articular fracture of the base of the thumb metacarpal.

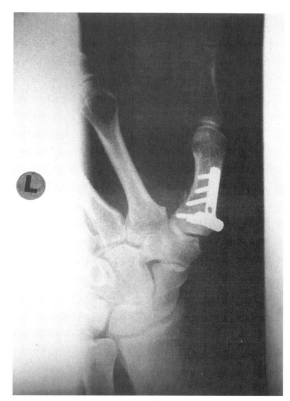

Figure 10.21. Rolando's fracture requires open reduction and internal fixation.

reduction is usually not achievable with this fracture which is usually managed by open reduction and internal fixation. Techniques of open reduction include: multiple K-wires, tension band wiring or plate fixation, using an L- or T-plate (Fig. 10.21).

Aftercare is as for ORIF following a Bennett's fracture.

References

Belsky, M. R. and Eaton, R. G. (1985). Closed percutaneous wiring of metacarpal and phalangeal fractures. In *The Hand* (R. Tubiana, ed.) pp. 790–5, W. B. Saunders.

Billing, L. and Gedda, K. O. (1952). Roentgen examination of Bennett's fracture. *Acta Radiol.,* **38**, 471–6.

Botte, M. J., Davis, J. L. W., Rose, B. A., von Schroeder, H., Gellman, H., Zinberg, E. M. and Abrams, R. A. (1992). Complications of smooth pin fixation of fractures and dislocations in the hand and wrist. *Clin. Orthop.,* **276**, 194–201.

Dennys, L. J., Hurst, L. N. and Cox, J. (1992). Management of proximal interphalangeal joint fractures using a new dynamic traction splint and early active movement. *J. Hand Ther.,* **5**, 16–24.

Duncan, R. W., Freeland, A. E., Jabaley, M. E. and Meydrech, E. F. (1993). Open hand fractures: an analysis of the recovery of active motion and of complications. *J. Hand Surg.,* **18A**, 387–94.

Foucher, G. (1995). 'Bouquet' osteosynthesis in metacarpal neck fractures: a series of 66 patients. *J. Hand Surg.,* **20A** (Suppl.), 86–90.

Holst-Nielsen, F. (1976). Subcapital fractures of the four ulnar metacarpal bones. *Hand,* **8**, 290–3.

Melone, C. P. Jr. (1986). Rigid fixation of phalangeal and metacarpal fractures. *Orthop. Clin. North Am.,* **17**, 421–35.

Meyer, F. N. and Wilson, R. L. (1995). Management of nonarticular fractures of the hand. In *Rehabilitation of the Hand: Surgery and Therapy* (J. M. Hunter, E. J. Mackin and A. D. Callahan, eds) pp. 353–75, Mosby.

Opgrande, J. D. and Westphal, S. A. (1983). Fractures of the hand. *Orthop. Clin. North Am.,* **14**, 779–92.

Pun, W. K., Chow, S. P., So, Y. C., Luk, K. D., Ip, F. K., Chan, K. C., Ngai, W. K., Crosby, C. and Ng, C. A. (1989). A prospective study on 284 digital fractures of the hand. *J. Hand Surg.,* **14A**, 474–81.

Simonetta, C. (1970). The use of 'A. O.' plates in the hand. *Hand,* **2**, 43–5.

Smith, F. L. and Rider, D. L. (1935). A study of the healing of one hundred consecutive phalangeal fractures. *J. Bone Joint Surg.,* **17**, 91–109.

Strickland, J. W., Steichen, J. B., Kleinman, W. B., Hastings, H. I. and Flynn, N. (1982). Phalangeal fractures: factors influencing digital performance. *Orthop. Rev.,* **11**, 39–50.

Further reading

Breen, T. F., Gelberman, R. H. and Jupiter, J. B. (1988). Intra-articular fractures of the basilar joint of the thumb. *Hand Clin.* **4**, 491–501.

Butt, W. D. (1962). Fractures of the hand. II. Statistical review. *Can. Med. Assoc. J.,* **86**, 775.

DeBartolo, T. F. (1996). Screw fixation of Bennett's fracture. In *Techniques in Hand Surgery* (W. F. Blair, ed.) pp. 265–73, Williams & Wilkins.

Freeland, A. E. and Benoist, L. A. (1994). Open reduction and internal fixation method for fractures at the proximal interphalangeal joint. *Hand Clin.,* **10**, 239–50.

Gonzalez, M. H., Igram, C. M. and Hall, R. F. (1995). Intramedullary nailing of proximal phalangeal fractures. *J. Hand Surg.,* **20A**, 808–812.

Hargreaves, I. C. (1997). Open reduction and internal fixation of metacarpals and phalanges. In *Atlas of Hand Surgery* (W. Bruce Conolly, ed.) pp. 99–113, Churchill Livingstone.

Howe, L. M. (1993). Fractures of the hand. *Scand. J. Plast. Reconstr. Hand Surg.,* **27**, 317–9.

Jupiter, J. B., and Silver, M. A. (1988). Fractures of the metacarpals and phalangeals. In *Operative Orthopaedics* (M. W. Chapman, ed.) pp. 1235–50, Lippincott.

Moberg, E. (1950). The use of traction treatment for fractures of phalanges and metacarpals. *Acta Chir. Scand.,* **99,** 341–52.

Ouellette, E. A. and Freeland, A. E. (1996). Use of the minicondylar plate in metacarpal and phalangeal fractures. *Clin. Orthop.,* **327,** 38–46.

Stern, P. J. (1999) Fractures of the metacarpals and phalanges. In *Green's Operative Hand Surgery.* (D. P. Green, R. N. Hotchkiss and W. C. Pederson, eds) pp. 711–71, Churchill Livingstone.

11

Joint injuries of the fingers and thumb

Joint and ligament injuries occur most frequently in the proximal interphalangeal (PIP) joints of the fingers and the metacarpophalangeal (MCP) joint of the thumb. Joint injuries are incurred frequently during sporting activities. They are often regarded as trivial and by the time treatment is sought several weeks or months later, the sequalae of pain, deformity and stiffness have become entrenched.

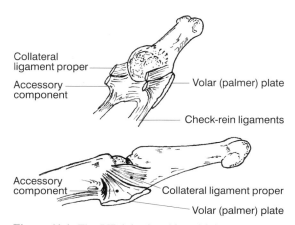

Figure 11.1. The PIP joint is a hinged joint with a flexion range of approximately 100 degrees. The thick collateral ligaments have a proper and an accessory component that are distinguished by their points of insertion. The collateral ligaments are the primary restraints to radial and ulnar joint deviation. The volar plate forms the floor of the joint and is suspended laterally by the collateral ligaments.

Anatomy of the PIP joint

The PIP joint is a ginglymus (or hinged) joint which moves in the sagittal plane and has a flexion range of approximately 100 degrees (Eaton, 1995). The joint is comprised of three main anatomic components: bone, ligament and tendon (Fig. 11.1).

The head of the proximal phalanx is a convex bicondylar surface with an intercondylar groove that articulates with the biconcave base and intercondylar ridge of the middle phalanx. The articular surface extends further palmarly than dorsally, thereby favouring flexion. The width of the joint is twice its vertical height and this contributes significantly to joint stability.

The articular surfaces, whilst mirroring one another, are not fully congruous. This lack of complete congruity allows slight lateral and rotational motion. When the PIP joint is flexed to 90 degrees and the proximal phalanx is viewed end-on, it is noted to have a trapezoidal shape; this shape varies from digit to digit. Combined with the accessory movements, these slight variations in shape allow the digits to adapt to irregular shapes when power grip is applied (Fig. 11.2).

The support system of the PIP joint

Capsular support for the PIP joint consists of tough collateral-accessory ligaments on the lateral aspect of the joint and a fibrous plate on the volar aspect. The collateral ligaments are 2–3 mm thick and are

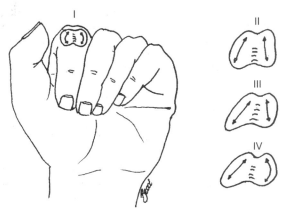

Figure 11.2. When the PIP joint is flexed to 90 degrees and the proximal phalanx is viewed end-on, it is noted to have a trapezoidal shape. This shape varies from digit to digit. This variation, combined with the slight lack of joint congruity that facilitates lateral and rotational motion, allows the digits to adapt to irregular shapes when power grip is applied.

the major restraint to lateral stress (Kiefhaber et al., 1986). They arise from the condyles of the proximal phalanx and pass in an oblique and volar direction. The collateral ligament proper inserts on the volar base of the middle phalanx while the accessory portion of the ligament attaches to and suspends the volar plate and tendon sheath. This latter portion is the more flexible and concertinas in the end range of flexion.

The volar plate forms the floor of the joint. Distally it is a dense fibrocartilaginous structure with periosteal attachment at the central base of the middle phalanx and dense lateral attachments at the corners. The thickness of the distal volar plate increases the mechanical advantage of the flexor tendons in the initiation of interphalangeal joint flexion. Proximally the volar plate is much like an inverted 'U' and resembles a swallow's tail. The two 'tails' are check-rein ligaments and are firmly anchored to the volar periosteum of the proximal phalanx. They prevent hyperextension of the joint yet are sufficiently flexible to fold upon themselves during maximum joint flexion.

The proximal end of the volar plate has a central membranous portion which bridges the retro-condylar recess. It is here that the major vincular systems to the flexor tendons originate. When the PIP joint is fully flexed, the base of the middle phalanx sits firmly in this recess, providing maximum stability. Obliteration of this space by

scar, bone spur, adherence of the volar plate or prolonged immobilization will produce a major restriction to joint motion.

Support to the dorsum of the joint is minimal, consisting mostly of the thin, semi-elastic extensor mechanism as it blends with the delicate dorsal capsule. Supplementary joint stability is provided by the lateral bands, the transverse retinacular ligament and the oblique retinacular ligament.

Signs and symptoms of PIP joint injury

1. Swelling.
2. Deformity (usually PIP joint flexion deformity) (Fig. 11.3).
3. Stiffness of interphalangeal joints.
4. Pain.

Assessment

1. History

The history should include the mechanism and recency of injury, e.g. did the joint dislocate laterally or dorsally and was it reduced at the time?

2. Physical examination

Observations during the physical examination should include: degree of swelling, type of deformity and restriction of joint motion. Acute swelling is usually soft and easily indented. When present for weeks or months it becomes fibrotic and results in periarticular thickening that gives the joint a fusiform appearance. The joint is gently palpated for specific areas of tenderness (Fig. 11.4).

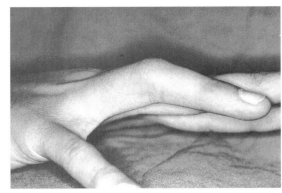

Figure 11.3. Injury to the PIP joint is invariably accompanied by a flexion deformity.

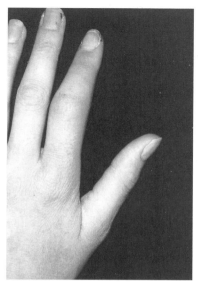

Figure 11.4. The injured PIP joint usually presents with soft swelling in the early stages after injury, and later with fibrotic periarticular thickening. Note the absence of skin creases over the PIP joint. Stiffness of both IP joints is common.

3. X-ray examinations

Posteroanterior (PA) and true lateral views of the hand should include views of the digit alone to avoid superimposition of the other digits.

4. Joint stability

If a serious fracture has been excluded, active and passive joint stability is assessed. Where the injury is acute and accompanied by pain, a metacarpal block will be required prior to this assessment.

Dislocation of the PIP joint

The PIP joint can dislocate dorsally, laterally or volarly. Most dislocations can be treated conservatively, the exception being an unstable fracture-dislocation.

Lateral injury to the PIP joint

Injuries to the collateral ligaments occur more frequently on the radial aspect of the joint and often have some involvement of the volar plate. They result from unilateral stress applied to the extended digit. A ligament injury can be regarded as a sprain if the injured joint has sufficient capsular support to prevent displacement under appropriate stress. If the lateral stress test produces a deformity of greater than 20 degrees, this will indicate complete disruption of the collateral ligament. These injuries are managed conservatively following reduction.

In the acute phase, these injuries are painful and accompanied by significant oedema which effectively 'splints' the joint in a semi-flexed position. While the oedema has some protective role, its prolonged presence will prevent movement and will result in adherence of joint structures.

Treatment

Oedema control and protective splinting

A single layer of 2.5 cm Coban wrap is applied to the digit in a distal to proximal direction. This is applied with great care to avoid lateral stress to the PIP joint. The finger is then rested in a thermoplastic finger splint in slight PIP joint flexion, i.e about 20 degrees if volar plate involvement is suspected or in maximum extension if the injury is regarded as a sprain of the collateral ligaments. The splint is worn for the first 3 to 7 days following injury to allow

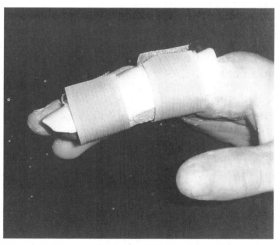

Figure 11.5. A single layer of Coban is applied to the swollen digit. A dorsal finger splint provides support during the first few postinjury days. If involvement of the volar plate is suspected, the PIP joint is placed in slight flexion, otherwise the IP joints are splinted in maximum extension. This may not be achievable on the first visit.

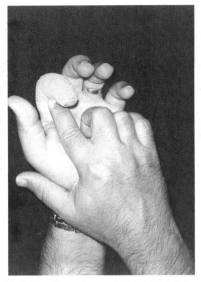

Figure 11.6. Hourly active stabilized IP joint flexion/extension exercises are performed through the Coban wrap.

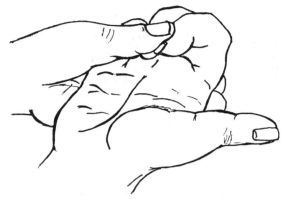

Figure 11.7. Intrinsic stretches are performed by holding the MCP joints in the extended position and gently passively flexing the IP joints. This manoeuvre maintains the length of the lateral bands and oblique retinacular ligament.

pain and swelling to settle. This period may be extended if there has been complete rupture and significant pain and swelling (Fig. 11.5).

Exercises

Gentle active stabilized IP joint flexion/extension exercises are then commenced through the Coban wrap. These exercises are performed on an hourly basis with 5 to 10 movements initially. As tolerance to exercise improves, the number of movements is increased. Movements are carried out gently and slowly and the end range position should be held for several seconds before the movement is repeated (Fig. 11.6).

Buddy-strapping

After the splinting period, the injured finger is taped to an adjacent digit to provide lateral support during activity. Coban wrap and Micropore tape are both suitable for this purpose. A buddy-strap fashioned from Velcro can be used if the joints of the two adjoining fingers are relatively level.

Intrinsic stretches

Adherence of the lateral bands or oblique retinacular ligament can occur following injury to the collateral ligaments. To help prevent contracture,

intrinsic stretches are incorporated into the exercise programme. The intrinsic muscles are stretched by holding the MCP joints in the extended position while passively flexing the IP joints (Fig. 11.7). This is followed by stabilized active DIP flexion exercises with the PIP joint held in extension; this manoeuvre places the oblique retinacular ligament on maximum stretch.

Overcoming PIP joint flexion deformity

The first line of defence in correcting and controlling a PIP joint flexion deformity is a neoprene fingerstall. The stall can be sewn in minutes and is easily applied and removed. It controls oedema, allows flexion and frequently reduces joint pain (Fig. 11.8). To gain the last 20 degrees or so of extension range, a Capener splint may be required (Fig. 11.9). Efforts to overcome the flexion deformity need to be balanced with consistent attention to regaining passive/active flexion range at both IP joints. The patient is advised to wear the neoprene stall around the clock other than when performing hourly flexion exercises.

Flexion strapping of interphalangeal joints

Where IP joint stiffness is marked, gentle flexion bandaging prior to active exercise is recommended. An IP joint flexion strap made from neoprene is used when the patient has achieved sufficient flexion range to hold the strap in place. Coban wrap (25 mm) or Microfoam tape also make effective flexion straps (Fig. 11.10). The tension of the strap

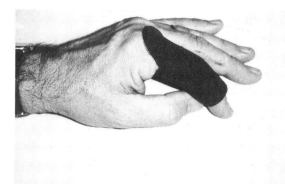

Figure 11.8. A neoprene fingerstall is the first line of defence in overcoming a PIP joint flexion deformity. As well as exerting a gentle extension force, the stall will reduce oedema and frequently relieve joint pain. Active flexion exercises can be carried out with the stall in place.

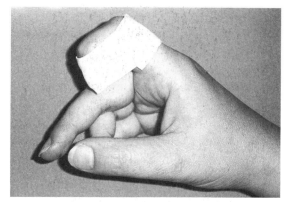

Figure 11.10. Frequent use of an IP joint flexion strap throughout the day will help restore flexion range. The strap can be made from neoprene/velcro, or alternatively, Coban wrap or Microfoam tape which is shown here.

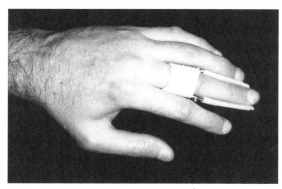

Figure 11.9. A dynamic Capener splint may be needed to overcome the last 20 to 25 degrees of deformity.

should be sufficient to provide a gentle stretch without causing pain or restricting circulation. It is left in place for 10 to 15 min every few hours during the day. Resisted exercises and activities are delayed until at least 6 weeks after injury.

Maintenance of home programme

Ligaments are notoriously slow to heal. Persisting pain, stiffness and recurrent joint swelling are common. The patient is therefore encouraged to maintain the exercise and splinting programme for some months following injury. Even when flexion range has been restored, the propensity for recurrent flexion deformity is great. Intermittent extension splinting by way of a neoprene fingerstall, Capener or static finger splint should be maintained until the joint no longer 'relapses' when

these devices are left off for several consecutive days. Use of the neoprene stall during the day allows unimpeded use of the digit. A Capener or static splint can then be used at night.

Dorsal dislocation of the PIP joint

Dorsal dislocation of the PIP joint is the most common dislocation in the hand. It results from hyperextension of the joint and is usually associated with a distal rupture of the volar plate from the base of the middle phalanx with or without an avulsed bone fragment (Fig. 11.11).

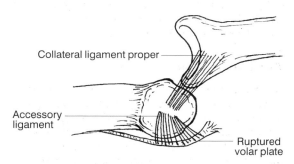

Collateral ligament proper

Accessory ligament

Ruptured volar plate

Figure 11.11. Dorsal dislocation of PIP joint. The collateral ligament proper remains attached and intact and usually provides stability after joint reduction. The accessory portion of the collateral ligament remains with the volar plate which ruptures from the base of the middle phalanx, either on its own or with a small avulsion fragment.

Treatment

The majority of these hyperextension and dorsal dislocations injuries can be reduced satisfactorily and treated conservatively. The PIP joint is splinted in 25 to 30 degrees of flexion for 1 to 2 weeks. Gentle active exercise is commenced 2 to 3 days after injury when the initial swelling and oedema have subsided. Oedema is managed with Coban wrap. Following removal of the splint, the digit is buddy-strapped to an adjacent finger for support. Extension splinting is delayed until the 5th week and consists of the same regimen as that which has been described for lateral joint injury.

Unstable fracture-dislocation of the PIP joint

Unstable fracture-dislocations are those where joint congruity has not been established following closed reduction or where more than 40 per cent of the volar articular surface is fractured (Fig. 11.12).

Surgery

Volar plate advancement (Bilos et al., 1994) restores a smooth fibrocartilaginous surface to the base of the middle phalanx. The joint is exposed and assessment is made regarding the possibility of reduction and fragment fixation. A single, large fragment can be reduced and held with one or two K-wires. Where the fracture is significantly comminuted, the fragments are debrided and the distal portion of the palmar plate is advanced 4–6 mm and sutured to the base of the middle phalanx using a pull-out suture. A K-wire holds the reduced joint in 25 to 30 degrees of flexion for 3 weeks (Fig. 11.13).

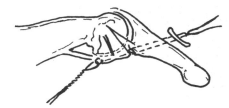

Figure 11.13. Volar plate advancement restores a smooth fibrocartilaginous surface to the base of the middle phalanx. The volar plate is sutured to the base of the middle phalanx using a pull-out suture. A K-wire holds the reduced joint in 25 to 30 degrees of flexion for three weeks.

Aftercare

Gentle DIP exercises are practised throughout this period. Following removal of the K-wire, the joint is maintained in the same degree of PIP joint flexion with a dorsal blocking splint for another week and gentle active PIP joint flexion exercises are begun. Unforced active PIP joint extension is then commenced at week 4. Any residual flexion deformity is overcome with gentle extension splinting from the 5th week onward.

Intra-articular fractures

Apart from hyperextension injuries, intra-articular fractures of the PIP joint (Morgan et al., 1995) can result from impaction injuries where the base of the middle phalanx is driven over the head of the proximal phalanx or pilon fractures where there is disruption of both the dorsal and volar articular

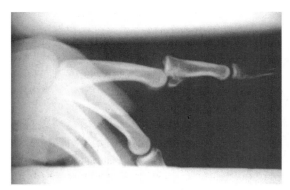

Figure 11.12. Radiograph showing dorsal dislocation of the PIP joint of the index finger with a significant articular fracture of the base of the middle phalanx.

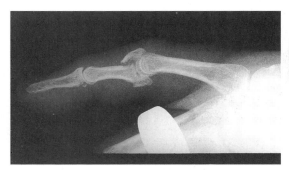

Figure 11.14. Pilon fracture of the left little finger sustained whilst playing cricket.

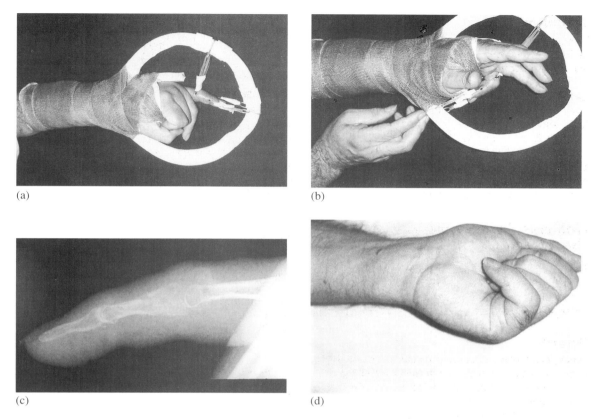

(a)

(b)

(c)

(d)

Figure 11.15. (a) The arcuate splint provides dynamic traction whilst allowing early movement. (b) Exercises are performed by the patient on an hourly basis. (c) Radiological appearance of the PIP joint at completion of traction period, i.e. at 6 weeks. (d) Active flexion range at completion of traction period.

margins and depression of the central articular surface (Stern, 1991) (Fig. 11.14).

Surgical management of these can include skeletal traction using an external fixateur or open reduction and internal fixation (Dennys et al., 1992) (Fig. 11.15). Treatment of these complex injuries has a significant failure rate and PIP joint fusion, implant arthroplasty or elective amputation may be indicated.

Corrective surgical procedures of the PIP joint

The most common complication of injury to the PIP joint is stiffness. Where adequate functional motion in either flexion or extension range has not been achieved despite a protracted splinting regimen, surgical release (arthrolysis) is considered.

Technique

This procedure is performed under selective peripheral nerve block. The joint is approached through a midaxial incision and the collateral ligaments and/or volar plate are released. If necessary, limited extensor and flexor tenolysis is performed.

Aftercare

Postoperatively the joint is splinted into the corrected position and active movement is begun within a day of surgery. Exercise sessions should be short and performed 1 to 2 hourly. Analgesia may be required for the first few days. Coban compression is used to control digital oedema.

Dynamic splinting is reinstituted after the first week when the postoperative soft tissue response has subsided. The tension of the splint should initially be low to gauge joint response. Dynamic splinting may need to be maintained for several months to prevent recurrence of the contracture.

Alternative salvage procedures include PIP joint arthroplasty or fusion. These procedures and their aftercare are discussed in the chapter on 'Arthritis'.

Thumb joint injuries
Anatomy of the thumb MCP joint

The MCP joint of the thumb has features of both a condyloid and ginglymus joint (Eaton, 1971). Its main movement is flexion-extension but it is also capable of some abduction-adduction and rotational movement. The thumb MCP joint differs from the finger MCP joints by having a radial and an ulnar sesamoid in the volar plate between which passes the FPL tendon. Unlike the finger PIP joints, the MCP joint of the thumb has no flexor sheath proximal to the volar plate and also has no check-rein ligaments.

Lateral stability of the joint comes from collateral and accessory ligaments. Volar stability is provided by the volar plate together with the thenar intrinsic muscles. Flexor pollicis brevis and abductor pollicis brevis insert into the radial sesamoid. Adductor pollicis and the first palmar interosseous insert into the ulnar sesamoid (Kaplan and Riordan, 1984).

Ulnar collateral ligament injury

This injury is commonly referred to as 'skier's thumb' and results from forced abduction of the MCP joint. The ulnar collateral ligament (UCL) is injured 10 times more frequently than the radial collateral ligament (Moberg and Stener, 1953). Distal tears at the insertion of the ligament are more common than proximal tears. Injury to UCL may be associated with an avulsion fracture where the ligament inserts onto the ulnar base of the proximal phalanx. It is important to distinguish between a partial and complete ligament rupture (Stener lesion). Where the rupture is complete, interposition of the adductor expansion will prevent the avulsed ligament from making contact with the rupture site, thereby impeding ligament healing.

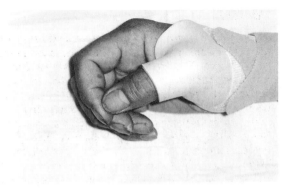

Figure 11.16. Partial tears of the ulnar collateral ligament are managed with a hand-based thumb splint which holds the MCP joint in slight ulnar deviation and flexion.

Diagnosis

Diagnosis is generally made on a clinical basis, although diagnostic ultrasound and MRI (Harammati et al., 1995) can help confirm the diagnosis where necessary. Signs and symptoms of UCL injury include bruising, tenderness and swelling along the ulnar border of the joint. Where 30 degrees or more of joint laxity is present, it is usually assumed that there has been a complete ligament rupture. Paradoxically, a complete rupture will often be less painful than an incomplete one. Radiographs are taken in 3 planes to assess the base of the proximal phalanx for avulsion fracture. Significant displacement will indicate retraction of the ligament and a large displaced fragment involving the articular surface will require open reduction and internal fixation.

Treatment of stable ligament injury

Partial tears are splinted continuously for 4 weeks in a hand-based thumb splint which holds the MCP joint in slight ulnar deviation and flexion (Campbell et al., 1992) (Fig. 11.16). Full mobility of the distal thumb joint is maintained during this time. Intermittent use of the splint is maintained for a further 2 weeks with the splint being removed every few hours for gentle active motion. Normal unrestrained use of the thumb is delayed until 12 weeks following injury.

Treatment for complete rupture of UCL

Because the results of conservative treatment for complete rupture are unpredictable, surgical repair is indicated.

Surgery

A 'lazy-S' incision is made over the dorsum of the joint. Care is taken to protect the superficial radial nerve. The adductor aponeurosis is identified and incised parallel to EPL. The articular surface of the joint is examined. If there has been a midsubstance rupture, a direct repair is made with interrupted non-absorbable sutures. Some distal ruptures can be attached directly to the remaining tissue on the proximal phalanx. Where there has been a small bony avulsion fracture, this is best excised and the ligament advanced to bone and anchored with non-absorbable thread or wire. A temporary transarticular K-wire is used if the repair seems a little tenuous. A large bone fragment is anatomically reduced and attached by pull-out suture, interosseous wire, K-wires or a small screw.

Aftercare

The joint is protected with a hand-based thumb splint for a total period of 6 weeks. The distal thumb joint is mobilized throughout this period to avoid adherence of the extensor mechanism. Splinting of the MCP joint is continuous for the first 4 weeks of immobilization. During the next 2 weeks, the splint is removed every few hours and gentle MCP joint exercises are carried out.

Unrestrained use of the thumb is delayed until 12 to 16 weeks following repair.

References

Bilos, Z. J., Vender, M. I., Bonavolonta M. and Knutson, K. (1994). Fracture subluxation of the proximal interphalangeal joint by palmar plate advancement. *J. Hand Surg.*, **19A**, 189–96.

Campbell, J. D., Feagin, J. A., King, P., et al. (1992). Ulnar collateral ligament injury of the thumb. Treatment with glove spica cast. *Am. J. Sports Med.*, **20**, 29–30.

Dennys, L. J., Hurst, L. N. and Cox, J. (1992). Management of proximal interphalangeal joint fractures using a new dynamic traction splint and early active movement. *J. Hand Ther.*, **5**, 16–24.

Eaton, R. G. (1971). *Joint Injuries of the Hand.* pp. 51–66, Charles C. Thomas.

Eaton, R. G. (1995). The Founders Lecture: The narrowest hinge of my hand. *J. Hand Surg.*, **20A**, 149–54.

Harammati, N., Hiller, N., Dowdle, J., Jacobson. M., et al. (1995). MRI of the Stener lesion. *Skeletal Radiol.*, **24**, 515–8.

Kaplan, E. B. and Riordan, D. C. (1984). The thumb. In *Kaplan's Functional and Surgical Anatomy of the Hand* (M. Spinner, ed.) pp. 116–7, J. B. Lippincott.

Kiefhaber, T. R., Stern, P. J. and Grood, E. S. (1986). Lateral stability of the proximal interphalangeal joint. *J. Hand Surg.*, **11A**, 661–9.

Moberg, E. and Stener, B. (1953). Injuries to the ligaments of the thumb and fingers. Diagnosis, treatment and prognosis. *Acta Chir. Scand.*, **106**, 166–86.

Morgan, J. P., Gordon, D. A., Klug, M. S., et al. (1995) Dynamic digital traction for unstable comminuted intra-articular fracture-dislocation of the proximal interphalangeal joint. *J. Hand Surg.*, **20A**, 565–73.

Stern, P. J. (1991). Pilon fractures of the proximal interphalangeal joint, *J. Hand Surg.*, **16A**, 844–50.

Further reading

Abbiati, G., Delaria, G. E., Saporiti, E., et al. (1995). The treatment of chronic flexion contractures of the proximal interphalangeal joint. *J. Hand Surg.*, **20B**, 385–9.

Arnold, D. M., Cooney, W. P. and Wood, M. B. (1992). Surgical management of chronic ulnar collateral ligament insufficiency of the thumb metacarpophalangeal joint. *Orthop. Rev.*, **21**, 583–8.

Bowers, W. H. (1981). The proximal interphalangeal joint volar plate. II. A clinical study of hyperextension injury. *J. Hand Surg.*, **6**, 77–81.

Dobyns, J. H. and McElfresh, E. C. (1994). Extension block splinting. *Hand Clin.*, **10**, 229–37.

Frykman, G. and Johansson, O. (1956). Surgical repair of rupture of the ulnar collateral ligament of the metacarpophalangeal joint of the thumb. *Acta Chir. Scand.*, **112**, 58–64.

Glickel, S. Z., Alton Barron, O. and Eaton, R. G. (1999). Dislocations and ligament injuries in the digits. In *Green's Operative Hand Surgery* (D. P. Green, R. N. Hotchkiss and W. C. Pederson, eds) pp. 772–808, Churchill Livingstone.

Green, A., Smith, J., Redding, M. and Akelman, E. (1992). Acute open reduction and internal fixation of proximal interphalangeal joint fracture dislocation. *J. Hand Surg.*, **17A**, 512–7.

Green, D. P. (1990). Dislocations and ligamentous injuries of the hand. In *Surgery of the Musculoskeletal System* (C. M. Evarts, ed.) pp. 385–448, Churchill Livingstone.

Heyman, P., Gelberman, R. H., Duncan, K. and Hipp, J. A. (1993). Injuries of the ulnar collateral ligament of the thumb metacarpophalangeal joint–biomechanical and prospective clinical studies on the usefulness of valgus stress testing. *Clin. Orthop.*, **292**, 165–71.

Inanami, H., Ninomiya, S., Okutsu, I., et al. (1993). Dynamic external finger fixator for fracture dislocation of the proximal interphalangeal joint. *J. Hand Surg.*, **18A**, 160–4.

Jobe, M. T. (1993). Fractures and dislocations of the hand. In *Fractures and Dislocations* (R. B. Gustilo, ed.) pp. 625–30, Mosby.

Mansat, M. and Delprat, J. (1992). Contractures of the proximal interphalangeal joint. *Hand Clin.*, **8**, 777–86.

Minamikawa, Y., Horii, E., Amadio, P. C., et al. (1993). Stability and constraint of the proximal interphalangeal joint. *J. Hand Surg.*, **18A,** 198–204.

Noszian, I. M., Dinkhauser, L. M., Orthner, E., et al. (1995). Ulnar collateral ligament: differentiation of displaced and nondisplaced tears with US. *Radiology*, **194,** 61–3.

Tonkin, M. A., Beard. A. J., Kemp, S. J. and Eakins, D. F. (1995). Sesamoid arthrodesis for hyperextension of the thumb metacarpophalangeal joint. *J. Hand Surg.*, **20A,** 334–8.

Wilson, R. L. and Hazen, J. (1995). Management of joint injuries and intra-articular fractures of the hand. In *Rehabilitation of the Hand: Surgery and Therapy* (J. M. Hunter, E. J. Mackin and A. D. Callahan, eds) pp. 377–94, Mosby.

12

The wrist

Peter Scougall

The wrist is comprised of several articulations, the anatomy and biomechanics of which are complex. Biomechanical interpretation has undergone some modification recently and continues to evolve.

Anatomy

The wrist is comprised of (Fig. 12.1):

1. The radiocarpal joint

At this joint the distal radius articulates with the scaphoid and lunate bones. This joint carries 80 per cent of the axial load of the forearm.

2. The midcarpal joint

The proximal carpal row, i.e. the scaphoid, lunate and triquetrum, articulates with the distal carpal row, i.e. the trapezium, trapezoid, capitate and hamate bones. The pisiform is a sesamoid bone that enhances the mechanical advantage of the most powerful motor in the wrist, i.e. flexor carpi ulnaris. The pisiform articulates with the triquetrum.

3. The distal radioulnar joint (DRUJ)

The head of the ulna articulates with the shallow concavity of the sigmoid notch at the distal radius. Twenty per cent of the axial load of the forearm is carried through the ulnar carpus via the triangular fibrocartilage complex (TFCC).

Radial tilt and inclination

In the sagittal plane, the radius has a palmar tilt of approximately 11 degrees. In the frontal plane, the ulnar inclination of the distal radial articular surface is approximately 23 degrees (Fig. 12.2(a)).

Ulnar variance

Ulnar variance (also known as Hulten's variance) refers to the length of the ulna relative to the radius. In ulna neutral (or zero) variance, the distal margin of the ulnar head articular surface is level with the medial corner of the radius. In ulna plus (or positive) variance, the ulna is 1–5 mm longer than the radius; in ulna minus (or negative) variance the ulna is 1–6 mm shorter than the

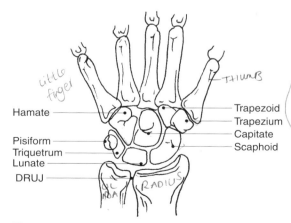

Figure 12.1. Schematic drawing of the volar aspect of the wrist showing the radiocarpal joint, the midcarpal joint, the eight carpal bones and the distal radioulnar joint.

When these movements are combined, a considerable range of motion occurs from radial deviation and extension to ulnar deviation and flexion. Range of motion can vary considerably among individuals. Wrist flexion usually ranges between 75 and 90 degrees, extension between 70 and 80 degrees, radial deviation between 15 and 20 degrees and ulnar deviation between 35 and 40 degrees.

Total range of forearm rotation is 150 to 190 degrees at the DRUJ proper and 260 degrees at the hand. Forearm supination and pronation ranges between 80 to 90 degrees when assessed from the midrange position with the elbow flexed to 90 degrees.

During wrist extension, the first two thirds of movement occur at the radiocarpal joint, the remaining third at the midcarpal joint. During wrist flexion, the first half of motion occurs at the midcarpal joint and the second half at the radiocarpal joint. Radial and ulnar deviation occur primarily at the radiocarpal joint.

Assessment of the wrist

1. History

Assessment is made of the mechanism of injury and the force involved. Was the injury associated with a 'snapping' or 'popping' sound or sensation? Does the wrist 'give way' during activity? Where and when is pain present? What factors aggravate or relieve pain? Note should be taken of the patient's expectations and physical demands in relation to occupation, sporting and leisure pursuits.

2. Examination

Look for swelling or deformity. Ask the patient to point to the most painful area; this area is palpated last. Compare range of motion and grip strength with the contralateral side. Check for generalized ligamentous laxity and perform specific tests to assess stability, e.g. the Watson scaphoid shift test, where appropriate.

3. Investigations

(i) X-rays
Many injuries can be diagnosed by plain X-rays. Special views may need to be requested, depending on the suspected pathology (see each section for details). If the diagnosis remains unclear after thorough clinical assessment and plain X-ray, other investigations can be useful.

(ii) Bone scan
This is a sensitive although non-specific investigation for suspected bone injury. Two days after injury, plain X-rays can appear normal while a bone scan will be positive, e.g. fracture of the scaphoid.

(iii) Tomography
Tomography can define the anatomy of the injury more accurately than plain X-ray. Bone healing and fracture non-union is more apparent than on plain X-ray, particularly where the scaphoid or hook of hamate are involved.

(iv) Magnetic resonance imaging (MRI)
Magnetic resonance imaging can be used to assess certain ligament injuries and is the best investigation for the assessment of bone vascularity, e.g. Kienboeck's disease.

(v) Arthroscopy
Arthroscopy has become an increasingly useful tool in recent years for the assessment and treatment of many wrist conditions including ligament injuries, articular cartilage defects and intra-articular fractures.

Fractures of the distal radius

Fracture of the distal radius is a common and often complex injury. The ultimate functional result will depend on accurate anatomic reduction. Unless this can be achieved and maintained, problems such as malunion, angulation, shortening and loss of radial tilt will result in wrist pain, stiffness, weakness and finally, post-traumatic arthritis. Incongruity or instability of the DRUJ or ulnar impaction syndrome are other potential problems.

Factors affecting outcome

Outcome will also be influenced by the patient's age and health status. A low velocity fracture in an elderly person with osteoporosis is a completely different injury to a high speed, comminuted fracture involving young, strong bone. Over-enthusiastic treatment of the first can be just as detrimental as 'under-treatment' of the second. The choice of treatment will depend on the individual requirements of the patient and the complexity of the injury. Fractures in older patients are generally treated less 'aggressively' than those in young adults although treatment decisions should be based on the physical requirements of the patient rather than simply on age. Severe osteoporosis and serious illness do, however, mitigate against an enthusiastic operative approach.

Assessment of distal radial fractures

1. History

How did the injury occur and what force was involved? High velocity injuries, e.g. falls from a height or from a motorbike at speed, involve greater soft tissue swelling and a higher risk of associated injuries.

2. Soft tissues

Open fractures require urgent surgical debridement. Acute carpal tunnel syndrome may occur and occasionally, the median nerve may even be divided. Ulnar nerve injury is rare. Tendon injuries are possible. Vascular injuries are rare after distal radial fractures, as is compartment syndrome (although this can be caused by a cast which is too tight).

3. The fracture

Adequate X-ray views are essential (posterior-anterior, lateral and oblique views). The opposite wrist is X-rayed for comparison. A CT scan may define the anatomy of intra-articular fractures better than plain films.

4. The patient

The treatment plan must take into consideration the age, general health, occupation, activity level, expectations and hobbies of the patient.

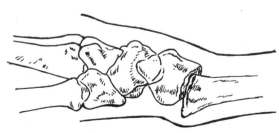

Figure 12.6. Colles' fracture with dorsal tilt of the distal fragment (Frykman, G. K. and Kropp, W. E. Fractures and traumatic conditions of the wrist. 1995. In *Rehabilitation of the Hand: Surgery and Therapy* (J. M. Hunter, E. J. Mackin and A. D. Callahan, eds) p. 320, Mosby, with permission.)

Classification of distal radial fractures

The more commonly used eponyms for the classification of distal radial fractures include:

1. Colles' fracture

This describes a transverse extra-articular fracture of the distal radius less than 2.5 cm from the wrist. The distal fragment is shifted and tilted dorsally and radially. It is usually impacted. The ulnar styloid process may be avulsed (Fig. 12.6).

2. Smith's fracture

This is a true reversed Colles' fracture, i.e. extra-articular distal radial fracture with volar shift and tilt (Fig. 12.7).

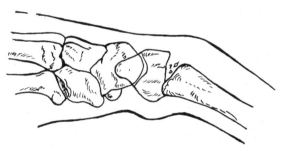

Figure 12.7. Smith's fracture with volar tilt of the distal fragment (Frykman, G. K. and Kropp, W. E. Fractures and traumatic conditions of the wrist. 1995. In *Rehabilitation of the Hand: Surgery and Therapy* (J. M. Hunter, E. J. Mackin and A. D. Callahan, eds) p. 322, Mosby, with permission.)

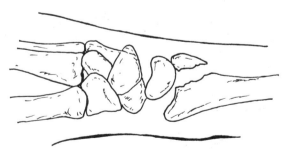

Figure 12.8. Barton's fracture-dislocation (dorsal). This is an intra-articular unstable fracture with either volar or dorsal fragment displacement. (Frykman, G. K. and Kropp, W. E. Fractures and traumatic conditions of the wrist. 1995. In *Rehabilitation of the Hand: Surgery and Therapy* (J. M. Mackin and A. D. Callahan, eds) p. 322, Mosby, with permission.)

3. Barton's fracture-dislocation

This is an intra-articular unstable injury. The carpus displaces with the articular fracture fragment. This fracture can be volar or dorsal.

Numerical classification

Contemporary authors prefer to classify fractures of the distal radius numerically. The higher the numerical rating, the more serious the injury and

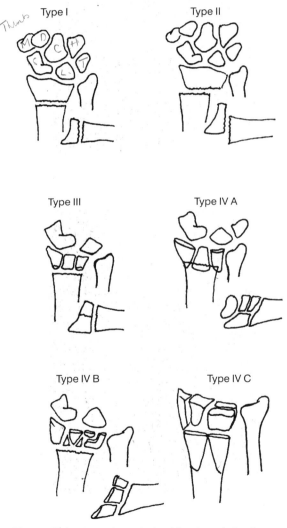

Figure 12.9. The universal classification of distal radial fractures as proposed by Cooney et al. (Cooney, W. P., Agee, J. M., Hastings, H., et al. Symposium: Management of intra-articular fractures of the distal radius. *Contemp. Orthop.* 21, 71–104, 1990, Bobit Publishing Co., with permission).

the more uncertain the outcome. These classifications are determined by whether:

(i)   The fracture is open or closed.
(ii)   It is displaced or undisplaced.
(iii) It is comminuted or non-comminuted.
(iv)   It is extra-articular or intra-articular.
(v)   The patient is an adult or a child.

Unlike earlier descriptions of radial fractures, these classifications include the ulna and DRUJ.

Some of the authors who have described classification systems include: Frykman, Melone, Rayhack, Fernandez and Cooney et al. (1990) whose classification is shown below:

> Type I – non-articular, undisplaced.
> Type II – non-articular displaced.
> Type III – intra-articular, undisplaced.
> Type IVA – intra-articular, displaced, reducible, stable.
> Type IVB – intra-articular, displaced, reducible, unstable.
> Type IVC – intra-articular, irreducible (Fig. 12.9).

Treatment of distal radial fractures

1. Closed reduction and plaster immobilization

Many fractures of the distal radius can be treated by closed reduction and plaster, particularly those that are low velocity, relatively stable and extra-articular, i.e. Types 1, 2 and 3.

A well-moulded plaster slab is applied initially. A short arm plaster is usually adequate. It should finish just proximal to the distal palmar crease to allow unimpeded flexion of the MCP joints. The limb is elevated and finger, thumb, elbow and shoulder movements are commenced. The cast is reinforced or tightened as needed and is completed when swelling has settled. The position is checked with regular X-rays. Gentle wrist movements are commenced when the plaster is removed; this is usually at 6 weeks (see p. 152 for therapy).

2. Closed reduction and percutaneous K-wire fixation (Fig. 12.10)

Oblique or comminuted fractures are unstable and likely to redisplace unless internally fixed. Closed reduction and percutaneous K-wire fixation is useful for extra-articular, incomplete articular and radial shear fractures if an acceptable reduction is achieved following closed manipulation. Great

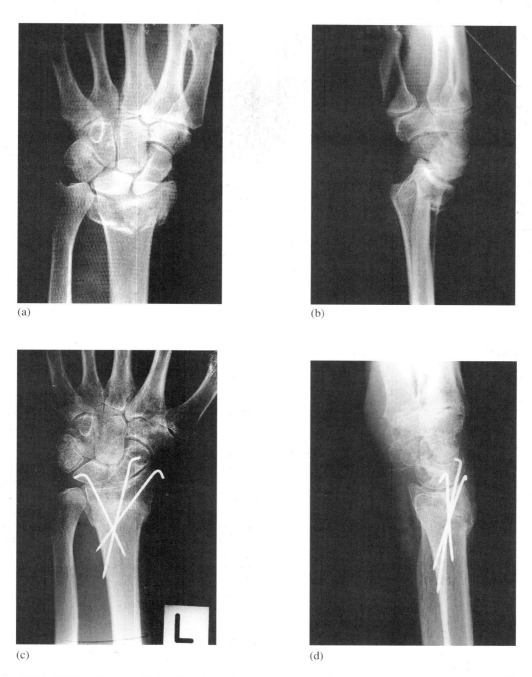

(a)

(b)

(c)

(d)

Figure 12.10. (a) This 63-year-old female sustained a low velocity Colles' fracture resulting from a fall while playing tennis. (b) Lateral view of fracture. (c) This fracture was treated with closed reduction and percutaneous K-wire fixation. Note restoration of the distal radioulnar joint. (d) Lateral view following closed reduction and percutaneous K-wire fixation.

care is taken to avoid damage to tendons, sensory nerves and vessels when inserting the wires.

The plaster is removed at 6 weeks and wrist movements are begun. The wires are removed 6 to 8 weeks following removal of plaster.

3. Open reduction and internal fixation

Open reduction and internal fixation (ORIF) is achieved with plates and screws and is indicated in the following circumstances:

(i)   A satisfactory position has not been achieved with closed reduction.
(ii) There is an unstable fracture pattern, e.g. Barton's intra-articular fracture-dislocation.
(iii) Displaced radial styloid fractures; these may be associated with scapholunate ligament injuries which should also be repaired.
(iv) Displaced or depressed intra-articular fractures, e.g. die-punch fracture (involving the radiolunate joint) (Fig. 12.11).

Metaphyseal bone loss should be grafted to prevent loss of reduction and non-union. Iliac crest bone graft is the graft of choice although various bone substitutes are available.

Aftercare

Open reduction and rigid internal fixation of the fracture allows early movement of the wrist which is protected initially with a plaster slab and then a thermoplastic wrist splint. The splint is removed every few hours so that gentle active wrist movements can be carried out. (See p. 153 for greater detail.)

4. External fixation

External fixation can be used to treat complex comminuted fractures or those with extensive soft tissue injury. Skeletal fixation via pins through the second metacarpal and distal radius allows precise, firm distraction of the fracture fragments (Fig. 12.12).

The technique is excellent for restoring length and radial inclination. Palmar tilt may be more difficult to restore and often requires an extra pin or K-wire. Displaced or depressed articular fragments may require open reduction via a small incision.

Associated soft tissue injuries, i.e. vessels, nerves and tendons, should be repaired at the same time as fracture fixation. Carpal tunnel decompression is frequently required.

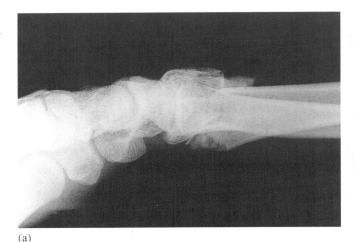

(a)

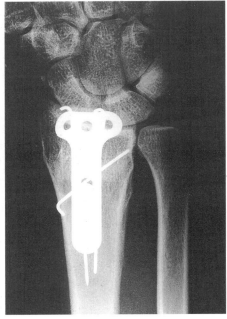

(b)

Figure 12.11. (a) This unstable comminuted fracture of the distal radius was sustained by a 28-year-old female who fell at high speed from a snowboard. (b) Treatment of this fracture required open reduction, cancellous bone grafting from the iliac crest and plate fixation.

The combination of oedema, wrist posture and restriction of finger movement due to the frame, can make finger flexion difficult. Composite flexion is usually not possible. The patient should therefore perform active intrinsic MCP joint flexion exercises separately to extrinsic stabilized interphalangeal joint flexion exercises with the MCP joints held in neutral extension (Figs. 12.13 and 12.14). Active exercises usually need to be preceded by passive flexion exercises.

Active finger extension is also restricted by oedema and tethering of the extensors. To help overcome this, 'place and hold' exercises are

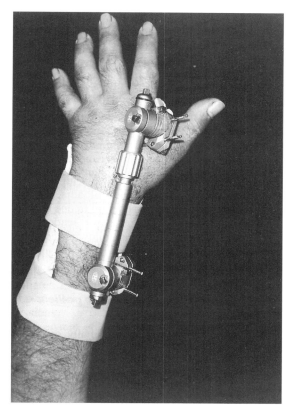

Figure 12.12. External fixation was used to treat this 32-year-old man's intra-articular comminuted distal radial fracture following a crush injury. Note the postoperative hand oedema which, if not treated promptly, will rapidly lead to stiffness of the finger joints.

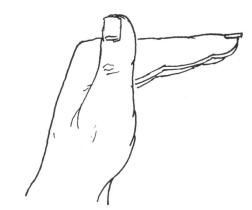

Figure 12.13. Active intrinsic MCP joint flexion.

Comminuted high velocity fractures of the distal radius can be difficult to treat and complication rates are high. Nevertheless, new fixation devices and better surgical techniques have improved the results of these complex injuries.

Therapy during fixator immobilization period

A thermoplastic wrist splint can be moulded around the frame of the fixator to provide volar support to the hand. Oedema, particularly on the dorsum of the hand, is often marked and can be addressed with light application of 2-inch Coban wrap. The arm should be elevated regularly and exercise of the proximal upper limb joints should be carried out frequently during the day.

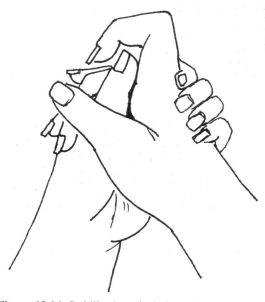

Figure 12.14. Stabilized extrinsic interphalangeal joint flexion exercises.

muscle-tendon shortening after protracted immobilization in a position of wrist flexion. Supination/pronation range is often quite limited.

4. Extensor tendon lag is common. Open reduction and internal fixation frequently results in tendon adherence (also known as tethering). The tendons can become adherent to one another, to adjacent bone or overlying skin. Rupture of the extensor pollicis longus tendon can be an associated complication.

5. The unsupported wrist is painful for many patients. This normal postinjury wrist pain is sometimes complicated by nerve involvement, e.g. an associated carpal tunnel syndrome or irritation of the radial nerve superficial branch during injury or surgery.

Hand bathing

Following cast removal, the hand and forearm should be given a prolonged soak in warm soapy water. The benefits of this are skin cleansing and pain reduction, particularly in the older patient. When the hand is removed from the water, the entire forearm is supported on a table, as suspending the hand in the air at this early stage causes discomfort to many patients. A rolled towel can be placed beneath the wrist in whatever position the patient finds most comfortable.

Oil massage

Gentle oil massage will help relax the patient, begin the desensitization process, soften the scar and assist with elimination of swelling when carried out in a distal-to-proximal direction. Warm water soaks and oil massage should be repeated several times a day as part of the home programme until the skin has returned to its pre-injury state.

Exercise

Exercise sessions during the first 2 weeks should be short but frequent, i.e. 1 to 2 hourly, and should not exacerbate pain. Before commencing wrist exercises, shoulder and elbow motion is assessed. The patient is reminded to incorporate all upper limb joints into their exercise regimen. Gentle active wrist movements including flexion/extension and ulnar/radial deviation are begun with gravity eliminated at this early stage. Active pronation and supination exercises should be performed with the elbow joint held in 90° of flexion; this position eliminates compensatory movements of the shoulder. To help isolate movement at the DRUJ, the patient should grasp a light object, e.g. a pen, to avoid using the finger and wrist tendons as a substitute for true forearm rotation.

Passive manoeuvres are used judiciously. Residual stiffness of the interphalangeal joints is overcome by bandaging the fingers into flexion every few hours to augment the exercise programme.

Hypersensitivity

Hypersensitivity that persists beyond the first 2 weeks or which interferes with the patient's ability to carry out their exercise programme is treated with transcutaneous electrical nerve stimulation (TENS). The patient should be issued with a unit for home use until hypersensitivity has resolved. This is usually achieved after 7 to 10 days.

Wrist support

The wrist may be splinted between exercise sessions and during light daily activity. This is particularly appropriate for patients who find it difficult to lift their hand out of the flexed posture because of pain, marked stiffness and/or lack of confidence. Serial extension splinting is instituted with these patients (Fig. 12.16). Intermittent support of the wrist has the following advantages:

1. Pain relief.
2. Helps resolve residual wrist oedema.
3. Overcomes stiffness when used serially.

While support splinting may appear to be a retrograde step following prolonged immobilization, the author believes that progress is expedited as the patient is more likely to use the hand when pain is reduced or eliminated. The patient is nonetheless monitored for a tendency to overuse the support.

Serial extension splinting of the wrist

The preferred material for serial wrist splinting is plaster as it gives a more contiguous fit and provides greater rigidity than thermoplastic materials. It is more comfortable in hot weather and is more economical where a series of splints is indicated. The close fit of the plaster, in combination with the compressive effect of the retaining bandage, provides good scar compression and

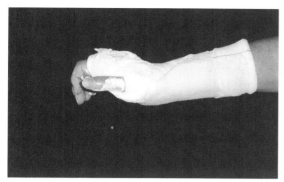

Figure 12.16. Serial plaster casting of a stiff, painful wrist will hasten progress by providing pain relief and increasing range of motion.

assists with the resolution of residual swelling. If silicone gel is indicated for scar management, the plaster is moulded over the covered gel.

The plaster cast should extend midlaterally on either side of the forearm and should attempt to hold the wrist in a slightly corrected position. Gains at each plaster change may only be modest; however, improvement in extension range over a 2 to 3 week period is often quite marked. The corrected position should cause only mild discomfort that usually settles quickly; it should not cause pain. The plaster is renewed every few days commensurate with improvement. The frequency of plaster change usually decreases after the first 2 to 3 weeks and is continued until a plateau has been reached, this generally occurring after 2 to 3 months. Progress is influenced by the complexity of the injury and the age of the patient. Discussion with the treating surgeon regarding realistic expec-

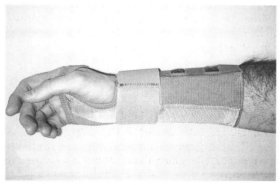

Figure 12.17. Where pain threshold is low or the patient is not confident enough to use the hand, the intermittent use of a soft wrist splint during activity can expedite progress.

tations is advisable. It is also important to stress to the patient that the splinting programme is complementary to their exercise and activity regimen and is not a substitute for it.

When a functional degree of wrist extension has been achieved, i.e. 20 to 30 degrees, a soft elastic wrist support can be used as an alternative during activity (Fig. 12.17).

Dynamic wrist splinting

Dynamic splinting of the waist is another option for overcoming stiffness; however, the outrigger portion of the splint can be impractical during activity. In the experience of the authors, the results of static splinting are equal to those gained with dynamic splinting.

Overcoming tendon adherence

Silicone gel compression and scar massage are maintained until scar has softened and tendon glide has been re-established.

Active wrist extension is synergistic with finger flexion. As wrist extension improves, there is a corresponding improvement in finger flexion. This is referred to as the 'tenodesis effect'. Conversely, active finger extension becomes more difficult as wrist extension improves, particularly when tendon adhesions are also present. To utilize the synergistic relationship between active wrist flexion and finger extension, early active finger/thumb extension exercises are best performed with the wrist in neutral extension or even slight flexion to take advantage of this tenodesis effect until the extensor tendons are less adherent and stronger. The wrist can then be brought into greater degrees of wrist extension during active finger extension exercises.

Tethering of the extensor pollicis longus tendon following ORIF can result in a lag at the IP joint. A mallet splint can be worn intermittently to prevent a flexion deformity at this joint. The splint will also assist in active thumb extension exercises. Where there is an extensor lag at the MCP joints, 'place and hold' extension exercises are preferable to actively extending the MCP joints from their relaxed posture of slight flexion.

Forearm rotation exercises

Patients often find it more difficult to regain forearm supination than pronation. Passive and active rotation exercises need to be practised as

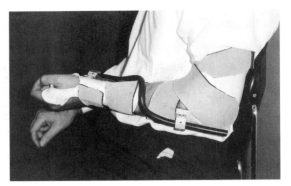

Figure 12.19. A dynamic forearm rotation splint is indicated if the exercise programme does not yield adequate progress in forearm supination/pronation range after a period of several weeks.

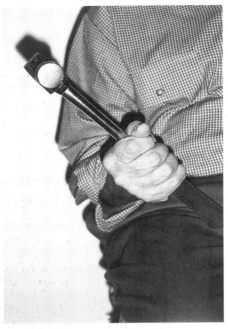

Figure 12.18. A hammer can be used as a passive weight stretch to increase forearm rotation. The weight of the hammer is readily adjusted by moving the hand along the handle of the hammer.

frequently as wrist exercises. Gentle stretches into supination should be maintained for short periods often throughout the day. Holding a hammer for short periods will assist forearm supination or pronation range by utilizing the weight of the hammer's head. The weight can be readily adjusted by moving the hand proximally or distally along the handle (Fig. 12.18).

Dynamic forearm rotation splint

If a satisfactory range of forearm rotation has not been achieved with passive and active exercise by the 6th week of therapy, application of a dynamic rotation splint should be considered. Approval by the treating surgeon should be sought before applying this splint as there may be contra-indications. The force exerted by the splint should always be gentle but prolonged. It is better to err on the side of caution and use too little force initially, rather than too much. The author has used the Colello–Abraham splint and the kit available from Smith and Nephew and has found both to be effective (Fig. 12.19).

Upgrading of treatment programme

Gentle resistance is added to the programme after a month and gradually increased over the ensuing weeks. Graded weights can be used to strengthen wrist flexors and extensors and the patient's activity programme is upgraded. The patient is strongly encouraged to use the hand and upper limb in suitable home and leisure activities. Where possible, return to the work environment is encouraged.

Cessation of therapy programme

It can be difficult to know just how long to persevere with the home splinting/exercise programme. A minimum of 3 months is usually required to attain a functional wrist range and reasonable grip strength. By this time the patient should have been weaned from formal therapy visits. Normal use of the hand will engender further mobility and strength. As a guide, formal exercise and splinting can be discontinued when active range of movement is equal to passive range and when there has been no increase in movement for several weeks.

Patients who are tentative about loading an unsupported wrist when they return to work are fitted with a neoprene wrist wrap. This allows unrestricted movement while providing support during activity (Fig. 12.20). Manual workers who place high demands upon their wrists can usually return to work at about 8 weeks following cast removal if good radiological and clinical union has been confirmed by the surgeon.

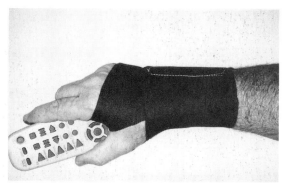

Figure 12.20. A neoprene wrist wrap allows full motion while providing firm elastic support to patients who are to return to heavy work.

Carpal fractures

Carpal fractures are common and often result from a fall on the outstretched hand. Their order of frequency is as follows: scaphoid, triquetrum, trapezium, hamate, lunate, pisiform, capitate, trapezoid.

Scaphoid

Fractures of the scaphoid represent just under 80 per cent of all carpal fractures. The scaphoid is the only bone to cross both carpal rows. Stress is therefore concentrated in its waist and fractures can occur with forced hyperextension. These are often high velocity injuries. The appearance of the X-ray will frequently belie the seriousness of the fracture. A fracture of the scaphoid waist requires twice the force necessary to fracture the distal radius. There may be other carpal fractures and associated ligament tears, creating instability and increasing the risk of non-union.

Blood supply to the scaphoid

Two thirds of the scaphoid surface is covered by articular cartilage through which blood vessels cannot pass. Scaphoid vascularity is therefore precarious and the bone can become ischaemic after injury. Eighty per cent of the scaphoid's arterial supply enters via soft tissue attachments along the dorsal ridge, derived from a dorsal branch of the radial artery; 20 per cent enters the volar aspect via the tubercle.

Clinical presentation

Patients with scaphoid injuries frequently present with wrist pain and swelling after a fall. Clinically, there is periscaphoid tenderness, particularly in the anatomical snuffbox. Range of movement and grip strength are reduced.

Diagnosis

The fracture may not be visible on initial X-rays, even when appropriate views are taken, i.e. PA view in ulnar and radial deviation (with the fist clenched), 45 degree oblique and lateral. The opposite wrist is X-rayed for comparison. If there is any doubt about the diagnosis, the wrist should be rested in a splint and reassessed at 2 weeks with repeat clinical examination and further investigations (Fig. 12.21). Due to bone resorption at the fracture site, the fracture will become visible on plain X-rays at that time. If early diagnosis is needed, a bone scan 48 hours after injury will accurately identify occult fractures. False positives occur with a 10 per cent frequency (Fig. 12.22).

A CT scan may be useful for more accurate definition of the fracture anatomy (Fig. 12.23). It will also assess union and detect subtle injuries. An MRI scan is very sensitive in detecting scaphoid fractures and for assessing bone vascularity. These scans are, however, expensive and not usually necessary.

The diagnosis of 'wrist sprain' should be avoided. The injury should be regarded as a fracture until proven otherwise. A missed diagnosis and delay in treatment increases the risk of non-union, carpal collapse and secondary osteoarthritis of the wrist. Ninety-seven per cent of patients with established scaphoid non-union develop wrist arthritis within 5 years. This statistic becomes important when one recalls that the majority of people with this injury are young, healthy adults who are frequently athletes or manual workers. In these patients, inadequate treatment of a scaphoid injury may result in disabling wrist arthritis before the age of 30 (Fig. 12.24). Early diagnosis and appropriate treatment are therefore important.

Treatment

Conservative treatment is indicated for:

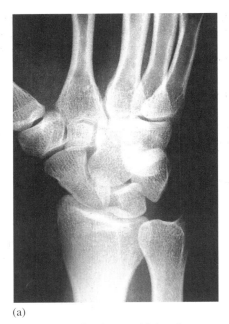

(a)

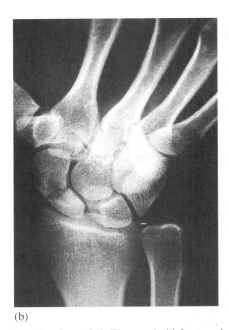

(b)

Figure 12.21. (a) This 19-year-old female presented with acute wrist pain after a fall. The scaphoid fracture is difficult, if not impossible, to see on this initial X-ray. (b) The scaphoid fracture is clearly visible on repeat films taken 2 weeks later.

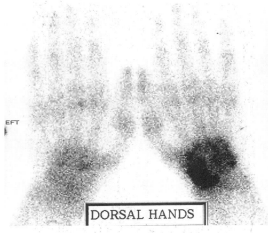

Figure 12.22. A bone scan can identify occult fractures 48 hours after injury if early diagnosis is required. This scan shows increased uptake in the scaphoid consistent with an acute fracture.

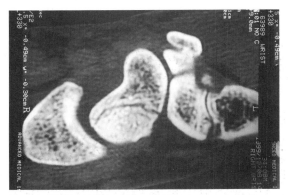

Figure 12.23. A CT scan can more accurately define the fracture anatomy as in the case of this scaphoid fracture.

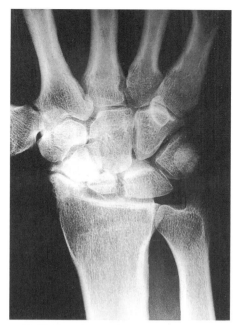

Figure 12.24. Post-traumatic osteoarthritis of the wrist due to an untreated scaphoid non-union.

1. Stable, undisplaced fracture of the waist

Stable waist fractures can be treated in a short arm cast including the thumb in a position of opposition to the index and middle fingers and the wrist in slight radial deviation and flexion (Fig. 12.25). Use of a long arm cast has been recommended by some to eliminate scaphoid motion due to forearm rotation. Recent experimental studies have shown, however, that such motion does not occur provided that the wrist and thumb are immobilized. Average healing time is 6 to 12 weeks, although this is frequently longer. Reported union rates vary significantly from 60 to 90 per cent.

2. Tubercle fractures

Tubercle fractures are rested in a wrist splint for 3 to 4 weeks. Waist movements are then commenced.

Indications for open reduction and internal fixation

1. Unstable, displaced waist fractures.
2. Proximal pole fractures.
3. Scaphoid injuries associated with carpal instability, e.g. trans-scaphoid perilunate dislocation.
4. Non-union.
5. Pathological fracture (Fig. 12.26).

The scaphoid is the most important bone in the wrist. The only acceptable result following acute fracture is solid bony union in an anatomic position. This is best achieved by treating unstable scaphoid fractures with early internal fixation.

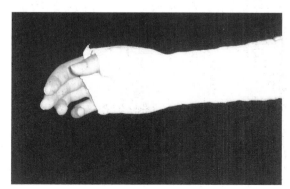

Figure 12.25. Short arm cast used to treat a stable scaphoid waist fracture.

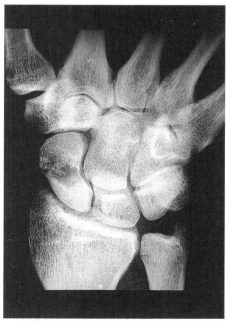

Figure 12.26. Pathological scaphoid fracture due to a benign enchondroma.

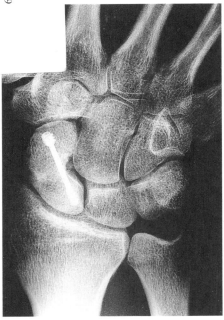

Figure 12.27. Scaphoid union following excision, bone grafting and Herbert screw fixation.

Advantages of early internal fixation include:

1. Increased union rate (90–95 per cent).
2. The avoidance of problems associated with prolonged immobilization, e.g. muscle wasting, joint stiffness, osteoporosis.
3. Rapid functional recovery with early return to work and leisure activities.

Technique

Fixation is achieved via a volar approach for waist fractures and a dorsal approach for proximal pole injuries. There are various fixation devices. The best, in the opinion of the author, is the Herbert screw.

The principles of surgical treatment are:

1. Debridement of the non-union to healthy bone.
2. Assessment of bone vascularity.
3. Correction of the deformity with a cortico-cancellous block of iliac crest bone graft.
4. Addition of a vascularized bone graft if indicated.
5. Rigid fixation using a Herbert compression screw (Fig. 12.27).

Postoperative management

Following surgery the arm is elevated for 24 to 48 hours. Finger exercises are commenced within a day of surgery. The wrist is immobilized in a soft bulky dressing or plaster splint for 7 days. Gentle active unresisted wrist exercises are then commenced.

Most patients regain good wrist motion within a few weeks of surgery and require little formal therapy once they are shown a home programme of active wrist exercises. Residual scar is managed with silicone gel.

The patient should refrain from heavy activities and contact sport until the fracture has united. This usually takes between 6 and 12 weeks depending on the size of the graft.

Salvage procedures

If the scaphoid cannot be reconstructed or the wrist has already developed secondary osteoarthritis, bone grafting and internal fixation are not appropriate.

Pain can often be controlled with non-operative measures such as support splinting and/or activity modification. If required, surgical options include:

1. Radial styloidectomy.
2. Wrist denervation.
3. Scaphoid excision and four-corner fusion (i.e. capitate, hamate, lunate and triquetrum).
4. Costochondral grafting (rib).
5. Proximal row carpectomy.
6. Total fusion.

Note: Prosthetic replacement is no longer used due to the risk of silicone synovitis.

Triquetrum

The triquetrum is the second most commonly fractured carpal bone, representing approximately 14 per cent of carpal bone fractures. Triquetral fractures are often associated with other carpal injuries and usually result from a fall on the outstretched hand.

Clinical presentation

The patient presents with pain, swelling and tenderness over the dorso-ulnar aspect of the wrist.

Figure 12.28. This 21-year-old man presented with ulnar-sided wrist pain due to a fall while skateboarding. Clinically there was local tenderness over the triquetrum. Plain X-ray had shown a large ulnar styloid process. This bone scan shows increased uptake in the triquetrum consistent with an impaction fracture.

Diagnosis

Triquetral fractures may be small avulsions, fractures through the body or impaction injuries, the last being the most common. The ulnar styloid is frequently longer in these patients than in the general population, i.e. there is an ulna positive variance. Diagnosis of these fractures can be difficult. Oblique X-ray views, CT or bone scans may be necessary (Fig. 12.28).

Treatment

These injuries will often heal if the wrist is immobilized in a splint or cast for 4 to 6 weeks in comfortable extension. If symptoms persist following non-operative treatment, arthroscopy may be indicated. This will often reveal an area of cartilage damage which can be debrided arthroscopically. Painful, un-united fracture fragments may require excision.

Lunate

Lunate fractures represent less than 2 per cent of carpal bone fractures and are usually associated with Kienboeck's disease (avascular necrosis). They are rare otherwise. The cause of this condition is unknown, although various vascular and mechanical predisposing factors have been implicated. Kienboeck's disease is more common in people with an ulna minus variance, i.e. the distal articular surface of the ulna is proximal to the distal articular surface of the radius.

The natural history of Kienboeck's disease is unpredictable and poorly understood. Ischaemia weakens the bone and allows it to collapse. While the ischaemia is reversible, collapse of the lunate and carpus is not. The purpose of treatment, therefore, is to correct lunate ischaemia early in order to prevent collapse.

Clinical presentation

The patient, usually a young adult, presents with wrist pain and stiffness often associated with swelling. Occasionally there are symptoms of carpal tunnel syndrome.

The onset of symptoms is frequently triggered by trauma. They may result from minor repeated trauma or occasionally, in a predisposed individual, from a single traumatic episode.

Diagnosis

The diagnosis is usually made on plain X-ray (Fig. 12.29). This will show lunate sclerosis. In the later stages there may be fragmentation and secondary wrist osteoarthritis.

Bone scan is useful for early detection and may be positive when plain X-ray is still normal. An MRI scan will also detect ischaemia early and may be used to assess the extent of the disease and the effect of treatment (Fig. 12.30).

Classification

Lichtmann's classification for Kienboeck's disease is widely used:

Stage 1 – normal lunate density; a linear or compression fracture may be visible.
Stage 2 – density is abnormal, i.e. the bone is sclerotic; no lunate or carpal collapse.

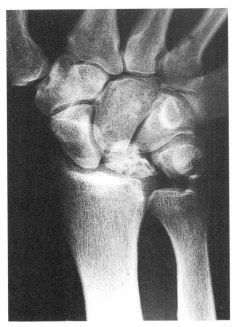

Figure 12.29. Kienboeck's disease showing advanced collapse and lunate fragmentation. Note the ulna minus variance.

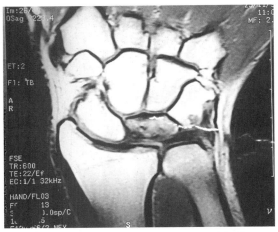

Figure 12.30. MRI scan showing Kienboeck's disease (avascular necrosis of the lunate). MRI is more sensitive for early diagnosis of Kienboeck's disease and can show ischaemia when a plain X-ray is normal.

Stage 3 – lunate collapse is present.
Stage 3(a) – carpal height is normal.
Stage 3(b) – carpal height is diminished.
Stage 4 – osteoarthritis is present.

Treatment

Treatment for Kienboeck's disease is influenced by the following factors:

1. The stage of the disease.
2. Ulnar variance.
3. Age and activity level of the patient.
4. The presence of arthritis.

Conservative management

Mild symptoms can be managed with intermittent wrist splinting, analgesia and activity modification. These conservative measures can often be used indefinitely. While there will be radiographic evidence of deterioration over time, more often than not, this will be unaccompanied by worsening symptoms.

The principles of surgical treatment

1. Reconstruct and revascularize the ischaemic lunate using a bone graft and vascular pedicle implantation (e.g. second metacarpal artery, posterior interosseous artery at the wrist).
2. Unload the lunate to facilitate healing.
   (i) In patients with ulna minus variance (Stage 1, 2 or 3), this is achieved by a joint levelling procedure such as radial shortening or ulnar lengthening.
   (ii) In patients with ulna neutral or positive variance (Stage 1, 2 or 3), midcarpal procedures such as scapho-trapezial-trapezoid (STT) fusion or capitate shortening are performed. Other techniques include dorsal capsulorrhaphy and radial wedge osteotomy.

Salvage procedures

If there is lunate fragmentation, carpal collapse or secondary arthritis, a salvage procedure may be indicated, e.g. proximal row carpectomy (if capitate and radial surfaces permit), wrist denervation or partial or total wrist fusion.

Hamate

Fractures of the hook of hamate are rare and represent less than 2 per cent of carpal bone fractures. This injury is associated with sports that

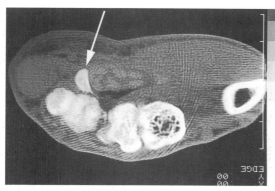

Figure 12.31. This 28-year-old golfer presented with pain on the ulnar side of the palm. Plain X-ray including carpal tunnel views appeared normal. The fractured hook of hamate is demonstrated by this CT scan.

involve gripping a club or racket (golf, tennis, squash, baseball or hockey) and is more common in athletes who grip the end of the handle in the palm.

Even when clinically suspected, this fracture may be missed as it is difficult to demonstrate on plain X-rays. Carpal tunnel views or CT scan are required to make the diagnosis (Fig. 12.31). A bone scan will show increased tracer uptake in the hamate.

Clinical presentation

The patient presents with deep, ill-defined pain over the hypothenar eminence. Symptoms are aggravated by gripping. There is local tenderness over the hook of hamate in the palm (2 cm distal and 1 cm radial to the pisiform). There may be ulnar nerve symptoms due to irritation in Guyon's canal. Active flexion of the little finger may be uncomfortable and flexor tendon attrition rupture can occur.

Conservative management

If the diagnosis is made early, the fracture may heal with rest and a trial of wrist immobilization for 4 to 6 weeks. This bone has a poor blood supply however and risk of non-union is high.

Surgical management and aftercare

Symptomatic non-union is treated by excision of the un-united fragment through a palmar incision, taking care to avoid damage to the motor branch of

the ulnar nerve. The bone surface is smoothed off to avoid irritation of the overlying tendons and ulnar nerve.

Postoperatively the wrist is immobilized for two weeks. A removable splint is then used and active wrist movements are begun.

Capitate

Capitate fractures represent 1 per cent of carpal bone fractures. These fractures may be associated with other carpal injuries, in particular, scaphoid waist fractures (scaphocapitate syndrome). This represents an incomplete form of trans-scaphoid perilunate dislocation. The treatment of choice is early internal fixation of one or both injuries.

The capitate is at risk of avascular necrosis because the proximal pole is entirely intra-articular. As with Kienboeck's disease, revascularization procedures have been used with variable success.

Postoperative treatment is the same as for scaphoid fracture following ORIF.

Carpal dislocations

Most major carpal dislocations result from a high energy hyperextension injury, e.g. falling from a height or a motorbike accident.

The two commonest patterns are:

1. Perilunate dislocation (Fig. 12.32).
2. Trans-scaphoid perilunate dislocation.

These injuries require prompt reduction. Both closed and open techniques have been used. In the

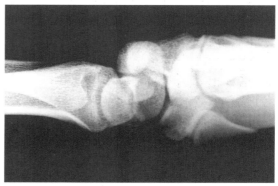

Figure 12.32. This 28-year-old man sustained a perilunate dislocation due to a heavy fall while playing rugby union. The scaphoid and capitate are displaced dorsal to the lunate.

opinion of the author, closed reduction and plaster immobilization are unreliable in maintaining anatomical alignment of the carpus. Open reduction is therefore preferred.

Surgery for perilunate dislocations

Perilunate dislocations are reduced through a combined dorsal and volar approach. The carpal tunnel is released, the carpus is reduced and ruptured ligaments are repaired. The reduction is held with K-wires.

Postoperative management

Postoperatively the wrist is immobilized in neutral for 8 weeks at which time the K-wires are removed. Gentle active wrist motion is then commenced and a removable splint is used for an additional 4 weeks.

These are major carpal injuries. The final range of wrist motion is approximately 50 per cent of normal and usually takes some months to achieve. It will take most patients at least 6 months (and often longer) to return to heavy manual work.

Surgery for trans-scaphoid perilunate dislocation

Open reduction is indicated for this injury and, at the very least, the scaphoid fracture should be internally fixed. Bone grafting may also be required if the fracture is comminuted.

Aftercare is similar to that for perilunate dislocation.

Carpal instability

Increased or altered carpal motion may occur as a result of:

1. Ligament tears.
2. Bony abnormality.
3. Ligamentous laxity.

If this altered motion causes symptoms, the wrist is said to be 'unstable' and treatment may be indicated.

Carpal instability can occur:

1. Between the bones of the same carpal row, e.g. scapholunate dissociation, lunotriquetral dissociation.

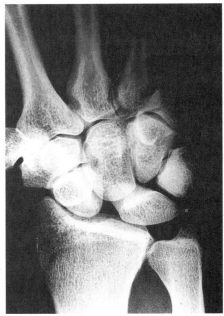

Figure 12.33. This 55-year-old man has a long-standing scapholunate injury. Note the increased scapholunate gap ('Terry Thomas' sign) and foreshortened appearance of the scaphoid giving a 'signet ring' appearance as a result of scaphoid flexion. Note also the early loss of joint space in the radioscaphoid joint. Arthritis begins here before involving the midcarpal joint. The radiolunate joint is usually spared (SLAC pattern).

2. Between the proximal and distal rows (midcarpal instability).
3. Between the radius and proximal carpal row (radiocarpal instability). This is often associated with rheumatoid disease (ulnar translocation of the carpus) or developmental Madelung's deformity.

Most midcarpal instabilities have involvement of both the radiocarpal and midcarpal ligaments.

1. Scapholunate dissociation

Scapholunate ligament injuries are a common cause of wrist pain and the diagnosis is frequently missed (Fig. 12.33). Untreated scapholunate dissociation will result in wrist osteoarthritis due to abnormal loading of articular surfaces, i.e. scapholunate advanced collapse deformity (the SLAC wrist).

Patient presentation

The patient presents with wrist pain and weakness, sometimes associated with a click or a feeling of 'giving way'. There may or may not be a history of trauma (usually a hyperextension injury). Instability may be associated with a dorsal wrist ganglion. Generalized ligamentous laxity is sometimes a predisposing factor. Patients with hypermobile joints are usually able to demonstrate the following:

1. Passive extension of the little finger MCP joint beyond 90 degrees.
2. Passive opposition of the thumb to the flexor aspect of the forearm.
3. Elbow hyperextension beyond 10 degrees.
4. Knee hyperextension beyond 10 degrees.
5. Forward flexion of the trunk with straight knees so that the palms of the hand rest easily on the floor.

Clinical assessment

There is periscaphoid tenderness, particularly dorsally over the scapholunate joint. Wrist motion may be normal although there is pain on full extension. Grip strength is often reduced compared with the opposite side. Generalized ligamentous laxity should be looked for.

The Watson scaphoid shift test (Fig. 12.34)

The Watson scaphoid shift test may be positive. This test can be difficult to perform and may be positive in normal wrists. Place the examining thumb on the tubercle of the scaphoid and the index finger adjacent to the proximal pole dorsally. As the wrist moves from ulnar to radial deviation, the examiner feels the scaphoid flex. Dorsal pressure is applied with the thumb on the scaphoid tubercle. If the S-L ligament is lax or torn, the scaphoid may sublux dorsally. This can be felt and may be associated with a painful click. Always compare with the opposite side.

Radiological examination

A thorough history and clinical examination will usually suggest the diagnosis which is best confirmed by arthroscopy. Plain X-rays are frequently normal, even if appropriate views are taken. These are: PA in radial and ulnar deviation, PA and lateral

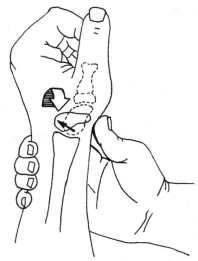

Figure 12.34. The Watson scaphoid shift test. (Reproduced from Garcia-Elias, M. Carpal instabilities and dislocations. 1999. In *Green's Operative Hand Surgery* (D. P. Green, R. N. Hotchkiss and W. C. Pederson, eds) p. 884, Churchill Livingstone, with permission.)

views in neutral. A clenched fist view may be helpful. The opposite wrist should be X-rayed for comparison.

X-ray signs that are consistent with scapholunate ligament instability include:

1. Increased scapholunate gap ('Terry Thomas' sign).
2. Increased scapholunate angle on lateral view (greater than 60 degrees); compare with the opposite side (Fig. 12.35).
3. DISI pattern (dorsal intercalated segment disability), i.e. the lunate is extended and the scaphoid is flexed (Fig. 12.36).
4. Foreshortened appearance of the scaphoid in the PA view due to increased scaphoid flexion; the scaphoid may resemble a signet ring.

The radiological features of scapholunate instability are frequently discussed but it is important to remember that instability, by definition, is a dynamic condition. Radiographs, even if 'motion' or 'stress' views are taken, are merely a static record of the wrist position at the time the picture was taken. Imaging studies frequently record fixed deformity, not instability. The instability grading system suggested by Herbert (1991) acknowledges the importance of clinical assessment.

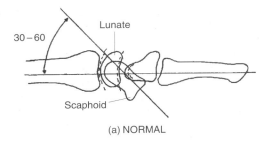

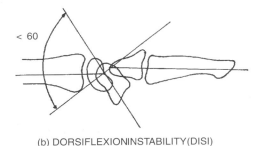

(a) NORMAL

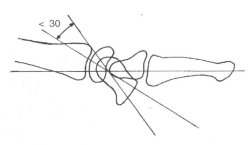

(b) DORSIFLEXIONINSTABILITY(DISI)

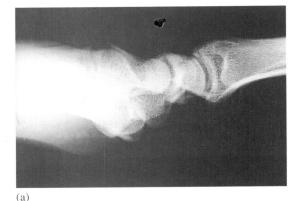

(a)

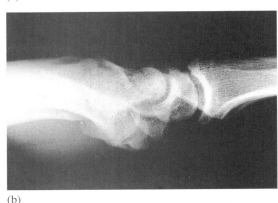

(b)

Figure 12.36. (a) This is the lateral view of the normal right wrist of a 22-year-old professional footballer. (b) Note the DISI (dorsal intercalated segmental instability) pattern on the injured left side where the lunate is extended and the scaphoid is flexed.

(c) PALMARFLEXIONINSTABILITY(VISI)

Figure 12.35. (a) When the normal wrist is viewed in neutral extension on a lateral X-ray, the normal scapholunate angle is from 30 to 60 degrees. Note how the long axis of the distal radius, lunate, capitate and metacarpal bones are collinear. Note also how the articular surfaces of the distal radius, lunate and capitate fit together like multiple Cs facing in the same direction. (b) When the lunate faces dorsally, the scapholunate angle is greater than 60 degrees (usually about 100 degrees). This angle indicates a dorsal intercalated segment instability (DISI). The capitate is displaced dorsally in relation to the radius. (c) When the lunate faces palmarly and the scapholunate angle is less than 30 degrees, this demonstrates a volar intercalated segment disability (VISI). (Reproduced from Frykman, G. K. and Kropp, W. E. Fractures and traumatic conditions of the wrist. 1995. In *Rehabilitation of the Hand: Surgery and Therapy* (J. M. Hunter, E. J. Mackin and A. D. Callahan, eds) p. 329, Mosby, with permission.)

Instability grading

1. Symptomatic wrist with no demonstrable clinical instability.
2. Clinically subluxable scaphoid.
3. Subluxed scaphoid, reducible.
4. Subluxed scaphoid, irreducible.
5. Secondary osteoarthritis.

Diagnostic assessment

An MRI scan can demonstrate partial or complete scapholunate tears. Dynamic ultrasound can show abnormal scapholunate motion when compared with the opposite wrist and will demonstrate an associated ganglion when present.

Bone scan is unreliable in diagnosing scapholunate dissociation.

Arthroscopy is the most accurate way to confirm the diagnosis. The ligament tear and abnormal motion are clearly visible.

Conservative treatment

Conservative treatment can be trialled with Grades 1 and 2. If the symptoms are mild or the ligament tear is partial, non-operative treatment is appropriate. A resting wrist splint is applied and resisted activities are avoided until symptoms settle. Gentle isometric wrist strengthening exercises are then gradually increased as comfortable. When the patient returns to heavy activities and/or sport, protective strapping or a splint is applied.

Surgical treatment and aftercare

For complete ligament tears, surgical repair is indicated. The malrotated scaphoid and lunate bones are reduced via a dorsal approach and the ligament is repaired with transosseous sutures. The reduction and ligament repair are protected with temporary K-wires (Fig. 12.37).

The wrist is immobilized in 10 to 15 degrees of extension for a period of 6 to 8 weeks. The K-wires are then removed and active wrist movements are commenced. A removable wrist splint is applied for a further month. Heavy physical activities are avoided for 3 months postoperatively.

Maximum wrist motion may not be achieved for at least a year. Wrist flexion range will be restricted to about 60 per cent of its former range.

Other surgical options include:

(i) Partial wrist fusion, e.g. scapho-trapezial-trapezoid (STT).
(ii) Ligament reconstruction using tendon or retinacular grafts.

As yet, no single technique has been universally successful in treating this difficult clinical problem.

Late presentation with established arthritis

Untreated scapholunate dissociation leads to arthritis resulting from the abnormal loading of articular surfaces. Cartilage wear begins in the

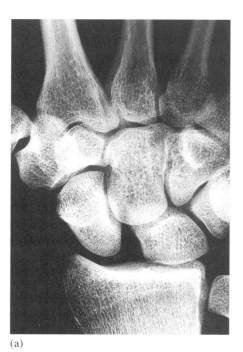
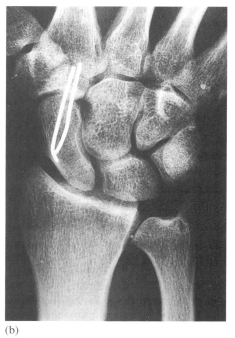

(a)   (b)

Figure 12.37. (a) Acute scapholunate ligament disruption. Note the widening of the S-L interval. (b) Ligament repair and reduction of malrotation. The reduction and repair are protected with temporary K-wire fixation (6 to 8 weeks).

ulna requires immobilization with the forearm in pronation. Dorsal dislocation of the ulna requires immobilization of the forearm in supination.

Stability of the DRUJ also depends on normal alignment of both forearm bones and integrity of the proximal radioulnar joint. The entire forearm should therefore be X-rayed. Instability associated with radial or ulnar shaft deformity should be treated by corrective osteotomy at the site of the deformity.

3. Triangular fibrocartilage (TFC) injury

Triangular fibrocartilage (TFC) tears may be degenerative or traumatic. Degenerative tears occur with an ulna positive variance and may be associated with other lesions such as articular surface wear on the lunate, triquetrum and distal ulna (ulnar carpal impingement syndrome).

Patient presentation

Patients with TFC tears usually present with ulnar-sided wrist pain that is often associated with a click. There may be history of a fall or twisting injury. Pain is aggravated by ulnar deviation and forearm rotation.

Diagnosis

The DRUJ is assessed for instability and increased carpal supination; comparison is made with the other side.

PA and lateral X-ray views are taken with the forearm in neutral rotation. Note is taken of the ulnar variance. An ulna positive variance may be associated with an impaction type cystic lesion on the ulnar side of the lunate.

Magnetic resonance imaging has an accuracy of 90 per cent in diagnosing TFC tears. Arthroscopy has the advantage of enabling treatment at the same time.

Conservative treatment

Initial treatment involves rest, immobilization and anti-inflammatory medications. If symptoms persist, arthroscopy is indicated.

Arthroscopic debridement

Central TFC tears are debrided arthroscopically. The unstable portion is excised and any associated articular cartilage wear on the lunate or ulnar head is also debrided.

Aftercare

Postoperatively the wrist is immobilized in a bulky soft dressing for 1 to 2 weeks. Gentle active wrist movements within comfortable limits are then begun.

(Note: Patients who have an ulna positive variance often require an ulnar shortening osteotomy in addition to arthroscopic debridement.)

4. Subluxation of the extensor carpi ulnaris tendon

Peripheral TFC tears may be associated with DRUJ instability and subluxation of the ECU tendon. Treatment for this involves arthroscopically assisted TFC repair and open reconstruction of the ECU tendon sheath if indicated.

Aftercare

The forearm is immobilized for 6 weeks in a sugar tong splint which holds the elbow in flexion and both the forearm and wrist in neutral. Gentle active forearm rotation and wrist movements are begun upon removal of the splint.

5. Ulnar carpal impingement

Patient presentation

The patient presents with ulnar-sided wrist pain which is aggravated by ulnar deviation.

Diagnosis

A plain X-ray (PA view) with the forearm in neutral rotation shows a long ulna relative to the radius. There may be cystic changes or sclerosis on the ulnar aspect of the lunate. The ulna positive variance may be developmental or acquired (e.g. radial shortening due to a malunited fracture, excision of radial head or premature closure of the radial epiphysis). The condition is frequently asymptomatic. Trauma, either a single episode or repeated minor trauma, may precipitate symptoms in a susceptible individual (Fig. 12.40).

A bone scan will show uptake on the ulnar aspect of the wrist. An associated TFC tear may also be demonstrated with MRI although this investigation is rarely required (Fig. 12.41).

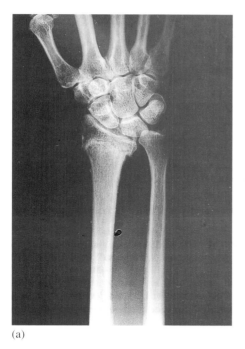 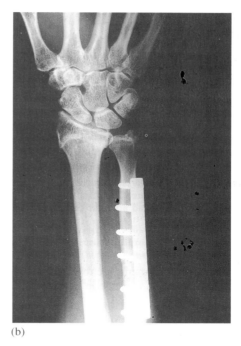

(a)   (b)

Figure 12.40. (a) This 52-year-old female had ulnar carpal impingement following radial shortening due to a malunited fracture. Note the ulna positive variance. (b) Correction was achieved by ulnar shortening osteotomy which restored the integrity of the DRUJ.

Conservative treatment

Conservative treatment involves a resting wrist splint and activity modification.

Surgery

Surgical options include:

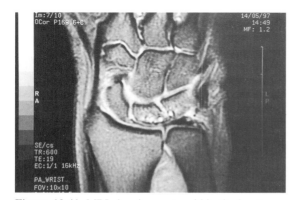

Figure 12.41. MRI showing cysts within the lunate and triquetrum of a 39-year-old female with ulnar carpal impingement due to ulna positive variance. This was also treated with ulnar shortening osteotomy.

(i)   Ulnar shortening osteotomy.
(ii) Corrective osteotomy of radial malunion.
(iii) Wafer resection of the distal ulna.

6. Osteoarthritis of the distal radioulnar joint (DRUJ)

The patient presents with ulnar-sided wrist pain which is aggravated by forearm rotation. The DRUJ is tender and irritable. The diagnosis is confirmed by plain X-ray.

Conservative treatment

Non-operative treatment involves splinting, non-steroidal anti-inflammatory medication and activity modification.

Surgical treatment options include:

(i) The Darrach procedure (Fig. 12.42(a))

This procedure involves subperiosteal resection of the distal end of the ulna (2 cm). Care is taken to protect the dorsal cutaneous branch of the ulnar nerve. The soft tissues, including the TFCC and sensation to the thumb is as important to function as is movement.

Other requisites of normal thumb function are:

1. Opposibility.
2. Stability.
3. Length.

Index finger

This digit represents 20 per cent of hand function and plays a vital role in precision pulp-to-pulp handling and lateral pinch. The musculature of the index finger is relatively independent and this helps contribute to its strength.

This digit provides stability and balance in delicate everyday activities such as writing and drawing. Length is vital to the index finger. As the level of amputation approaches the PIP joint, pinch grip function is automatically transferred to the middle finger (Fig. 13.3). Because of the impact on power grip associated with total loss of the index finger, every effort is made to conserve the proximal phalanx in manual workers (Murray et al., 1977).

Middle finger

The middle finger represents 20 per cent of hand function. In flexion, this digit has greater strength than the index finger. It is the longest of the digits and its central position enables it to participate in precision as well as power grip. Loss of the middle finger constitutes a greater aesthetic loss than that

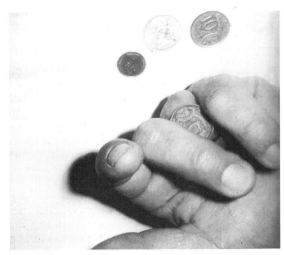

Figure 13.4. Loss of the ring finger allows small objects to fall through the hand.

associated with the index finger, as the adjacent digits tend to converge toward the residual gap.

Ring finger

The ring finger represents 10 per cent of hand function. This digit, together with the little finger, participates in strong digital-palmar grip. The ring finger is rarely used in precision grip. Loss of this digit results in the least functional deficit when compared to the other digits (Fig. 13.4).

Little finger

The little finger accounts for the remaining 10 per cent of hand function. The ability of this digit to abduct widely is of great functional significance in grasping larger objects. The gripping ability of the little finger is enhanced by its greater range of motion at the MCP joint where strength is reinforced by the powerful hypothenar muscles.

Psychological aspects

Wherever circumstances allow, the patient's emotional attitude toward amputation should be taken into account. Individual reaction to amputation is by no means always proportional to the extent of the loss. A patient who has lost the tip of a single digit may be as traumatized as another patient whose loss involves multiple digits. Pre-injury

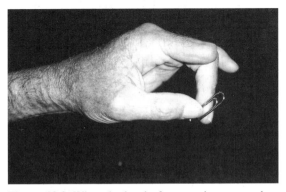

Figure 13.3. When the level of amputation approaches the PIP joint of the index finger, pinch function will automatically be transferred to the middle finger. In the case of this patient who has undergone elective ray amputation of his index finger and has a middle finger stump, pinch grip is transferred to the adjacent ring finger.

personality, attitudes and motivation will strongly influence a patient's coping mechanism (Grant, 1980).

Self-esteem relating to body image can be seriously damaged following loss of a part. Religious and cultural factors will often play an important role in the patient's reaction. Potential loss of employment as a result of the injury will have major emotional and psychosocial consequences. Financial consequences for workers with dependent families will be enormous if the individual is unable to return to pre-injury employment.

Whatever the psychological manifestation, it is important to afford it the same attention as the injured part. If there is any concern regarding the patient's ability to cope with the aftermath of the injury, referral to a social worker, psychologist or psychiatrist should be considered. Signs and symptoms of impending depression may include: loss of appetite, the development of sleeping problems, loss of interest in personal appearance, conversation that dwells on only negative aspects of the person's life or withdrawal from social activities.

Fingertip injuries

Digital tip amputations are the most common type of amputation in the upper limb. Management of these injuries includes: primary closure, split-thickness and full-thickness skin grafting, or advancement flaps, e.g. V-Y, volar or local rotation. Cross-finger pedicle or thenar flaps may be indicated for the younger patient with no pre-existing degenerative arthritis and in whom the development of stiffness is not considered to be a risk. Choice of treatment will depend on the degree of tissue loss, the presence of exposed bone and the personal preference of the treating surgeon (Fig. 13.5).

Problems associated with fingertip injuries

1. Hypersensitivity.
2. Altered sensibility.
3. Cold intolerance.

These problems are a result of the injury rather than the treatment and their incidence is significant in the adult patient with loss of pulp (Conolly and Goulston, 1973).

Therapy programme

Desensitization is not commenced until wound healing is complete. To help reduce pulp oedema and for the provision of comfort, dressings can be held in place with a lightly applied layer of Coban wrap (25 mm).

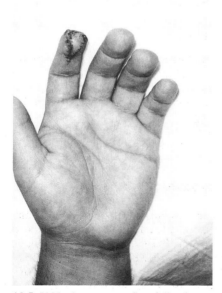
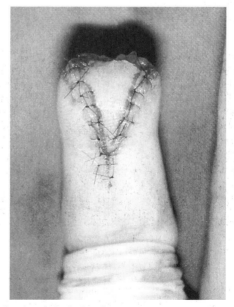

Figure 13.5. V-Y advancement flap following a crush injury to the tip of the index finger.

The patient is instructed in gentle passive/active interphalangeal joint exercises which should be performed frequently throughout the day. When sufficient healing has occurred, usually at 10 to 14 days, warm water soaks are commenced to debride the area in preparation for skin management and desensitization. Skin is then massaged lightly with oil. Massage pressure used can be gradually increased commensurate with the patient's progress. Short gentle percussion exercises are performed on an hourly basis. Most patients require very little formal therapy once they are shown a home programme of exercises. Patients are reminded to make every effort to incorporate the injured digit during activity.

Persisting hypersensitivity

Where fingertip hypersensitivity is extreme or persistent, the area can be covered with Opsite Flexifix. This usually reduces discomfort substantially whilst still allowing full sensory input. The film can be worn continuously and is reasonably water-resistant. It is simply replaced when it begins to lift at the edges. Opsite Flexifix can be used on its own or in conjunction with Coban wrap or a silicone-tipped fingerstall if scar management or shaping of the pulp are required (Fig. 13.6).

Surgical considerations for elective digital amputation

The requisites of a satisfactory stump include:

1. Adequate length.
2. Sufficient soft tissue cover.
3. Sensibility.

Surgical technique

1. Skin flaps of sufficient size are raised to expose the underlying bone, flexor and extensor tendons, and neurovascular bundles.
2. If the amputation is through an IP joint, the articular cartilage is not removed, but the condyles and any rough projections of bone are nibbled away.
3. Flexor and extensor tendons are cut so that they lie away from the stump. If they are sutured over the stump, they will interfere with the movements of the other fingers.

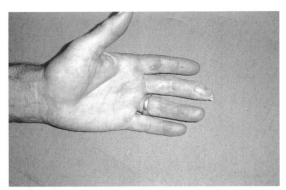

Figure 13.6. Opsite Flexifix applied to this skin-grafted middle finger tip significantly reduced hypersensitivity and allowed the patient to use the digit.

4. Digital nerves are dissected and cleanly divided about 1 cm proximal to the stump, so that any neuroma that forms is not at the scar line.
5. Skin is closed accurately and a non-adherent compression bandage is applied.
6. The wrist and digit are splinted in elevation for at least 48 h.

Possible complications

1. Poor skin cover.
2. Poor circulation.
3. Neuroma formation.
4. Stiff joints of the injured or adjacent digits.
5. Inadequate length for function.
6. Phantom pain (Jensen et al., 1985).
7. Dystrophy.

Postoperative therapy of digital amputations

The aim of treatment is to regain movement and function as quickly as possible. This is accomplished by a combination of passive and active exercise and desensitization techniques. Early function is also encouraged (Fig. 13.7).

The hand is rested in a light plaster and kept elevated for the first few postoperative days. Three days after surgery, gentle active stabilized flexion/extension exercises are begun. Full range of movement is maintained at all upper limb joints. Stump dressings should be minimal so that IP joint motion can be performed without the restriction of a too-bulky dressing. Coban wrap (25 mm) is used to hold the dressing in place, to treat pulp oedema and to help shape the stump (Fig. 13.8).

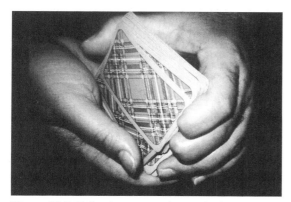

Figure 13.7. Following amputation, early function is encouraged.

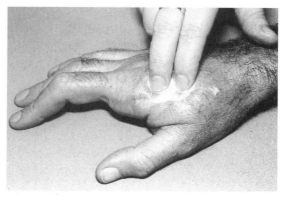

Figure 13.9. Oil or cream massage softens the scar line and is an important part of the desensitization process.

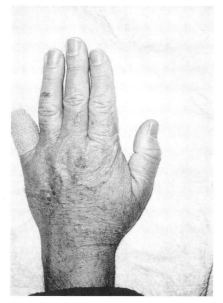

Figure 13.8. Coban wrap (25 mm) is used to hold the dressing in place, reduce pulp oedema and shape the stump.

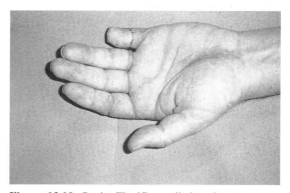

Figure 13.10. Opsite Flexifix applied to the stump significantly alleviates hypersensitivity. This makes desensitization exercises easier and encourages early function. The area of application is highlighted.

The hand should be used for light self-care activities as soon as possible. Early use of the hand improves mobility, assists with the desensitization process and has a positive psychological effect. Sutures are usually removed between 10 and 14 days at which time warm water soaks (containing a mild cleansing agent) are carried out several times a day. These will assist with wound debridement and help facilitate movement if stiffness is still a problem. Light sponge squeezing in the water will also promote movement and help with desensitiza-tion. Light massage with cream or oil will soften the scar and plays an important part in the desensitization process (Fig. 13.9).

Opsite Flexifix is applied to the stump to reduce sensitivity at this early stage (Boscheinen-Morrin and Shannon, 2000). Patients generally find their desensitization exercises much easier to perform through the Opsite layer. They are also more inclined to use the stump during activity when the film is in place (Fig. 13.10). Coban wrap or silicone-lined fingerstalls can be used in conjunc-tion with the Opsite for scar management and stump shaping (Fig. 13.11).

In preparation for return to work, patients are encouraged to use the hand for normal domestic and house maintenance activities. Carrying light shopping bags, hanging out washing, window

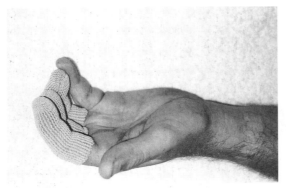

Figure 13.11. Silicone-lined mesh fingerstalls can be used over the Opsite film where hypersensitivity is severe or where scar management is still indicated.

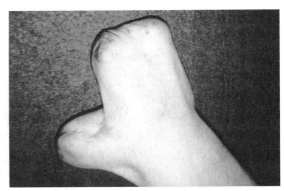

Figure 13.12. This 18-year-old apprentice carpenter was left with a 'mitten' hand following a circular saw injury at work. The re-creation of a thumb web restored gross grasp and enabled him to complete his apprenticeship.

washing, etc., will all help encourage normal use of the hand and entire upper limb. Attempting to use equipment such as vacuum cleaners or lawn mowers for short periods will help acclimatize the hand to vibration. Gardening activities will promote gross gripping and general fitness. Most patients are able to resume manual work within 4 to 6 weeks after amputation.

Reconstruction

Where replantation was not possible, reconstructive procedures can be considered. The patient's suitability is assessed in terms of age, occupation, leisure pursuits and hobbies, hand dominance, general health and the psychological ability to cope with sometimes numerous surgical procedures and aftercare programmes.

Reconstruction is most often used for restoration of pinch grip function. This can involve rearrangement of hand remnants or reconstruction of the thumb itself.

Local rearrangement of hand remnants

1. Deepening of the interdigital cleft, e.g. the thumb web, by Z-plasty lengthening of the skin and sliding the thenar muscle attachments down the shaft of the first metacarpal (Fig. 13.12).
2. Transfer of a digit, i.e. pollicization, when the metacarpal of the donor digit (e.g. index finger) is divided and transferred to the recipient stump; internal fixation is used to stabilize the transferred digit.

Toe to thumb reconstruction

Complete or partial toe transfer has proved effective in reconstructing the absent or deficient thumb. The toe has strong skeletal support, a nail, glabrous skin that can be reinnervated and mobile joints. Problems of size discrepancy (the large toe is about 20 per cent larger than the thumb) have been partly addressed with the 'wraparound' and 'trimmed toe' procedures.

While toe transplantation has the disadvantage of toe loss, the transplanted toe mimics the structure and function of a thumb more closely than any other thumb reconstruction procedure.

The five toe transplant options for thumb reconstruction include:

1. Whole great toe transfer (Fig. 13.13).
2. Second toe transfer.
3. The 'wraparound' procedure (Morrison et al., 1980) – this procedure is suitable for thumb loss distal to the MCP joint and involves transfer of a soft tissue flap and nail from the great toe; bony support is supplied by an iliac bone graft rather than the phalanges of the great toe. This transfer does not provide motion.
4. The 'trimmed toe' technique – the great toe is trimmed to the dimensions of the opposite thumb. Like the 'wraparound' technique, this procedure is used primarily for thumb loss distal to the MCP joint. Unlike the 'wraparound' technique, this procedure does provide motion.
5. Partial toe transplant.

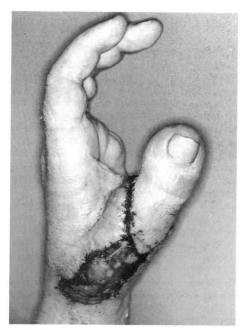

Figure 13.13. Transfer of the great toe to the thumb two weeks after surgery.

Sensation in the new thumb is anticipated in approximately 4 to 6 months.

Distraction lengthening of the metacarpals and phalanges (callotasis)

Distraction lengthening is a means of restoring functional length to a hand that is skeletally deficient through trauma or congenital absence (Seitz, 1999). This technique was first used for elongation of the long bones in the lower limbs. Although this procedure improves hand cosmesis, its primary goal is to enhance mechanical advantage and thereby function. This procedure requires high patient compliance; patient selection is therefore crucial.

Distraction lengthening can be applied to the thumb or multiple digital rays. A midshaft osteotomy is made through the metacarpals or phalanges and the distraction device is applied. The lengthening process begins on the 5th postoperative day for children and the 7th postoperative day in the case of adults. The process involves four daily increments of 0.25 mm each. About 2–2.5 cm of lengthening can be obtained through remodelling of the fracture callus. Following the lengthening period, the device needs to be worn for an

additional period to allow complete bony consolidation. The extended period needs to be 2 to 3 times the duration of the lengthening period and the device is not removed until there is radiological evidence of consolidation of at least three cortices.

Partial hand prostheses

Where replantation or reconstruction are inappropriate or rejected by the patient, a prosthetic aid, for function and/or cosmesis, should be offered to the patient. Immediately after surgery, the cosmetic appearance of the hand is of major importance to some patients, especially to women. Many will demand immediate fitting of a cosmetic digit. By the time fitting of the device can be arranged (i.e. often weeks postinjury when the size

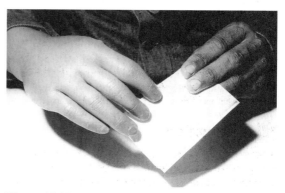

Figure 13.14. Some patients with significant hand loss wear a cosmetic prosthesis when in public.

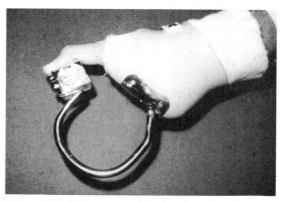

Figure 13.15. The most common types of functional hand prostheses are those which provide an opposition 'post' to enable gross pinch grip.

dorsum of the radius down to the third metacarpal. Cortical screws are used over the radius and metacarpal regions and cancellous screws help fix the carpal bones to the graft.

Aftercare

Fusion of the wrist is a major procedure which often results in significant postoperative pain and swelling. The patient should maintain bed rest and elevation for the first 2 to 3 postoperative days. The immediate postoperative plaster will need to be renewed at least once to accommodate changes in oedema.

The wrist is protected with a removable splint and movement of the fingers, thumb and other upper limb joints is commenced within a day of surgery. The wrist should not be loaded until there is radiological evidence of bony union, usually at 10 to 12 weeks.

Removal of the plate is an option but is delayed for 12 months until there is no doubt that the graft has consolidated and that fusion is complete.

Arthroplasty

The use of prosthetic arthroplasty spans almost half a century. Silicone elastomer implants (Swanson, 1968 and Niebauer et al., 1969) became available in the 1960s and despite problems with 'fracturing' and recurrence of deformity, the modified Swanson

silicone implant has been a reliable and accepted form of arthroplasty since that time.

Newer implants are currently being trialled. The 'Neuflex' silicone MCP joint prosthesis, introduced by Weiss, incorporates a flexed posture in the joint hinge which has resulted in improved MCP joint flexion range. Postoperative care is the same as for other silicone implants.

Linscheid has developed a new MCP surface replacement arthroplasty similar to that for the PIP joint. The proximal component is composed of a chromium-cobalt alloy and the distal component is made of ultrahigh-molecular-weight polyethylene.

Arthroplasty is the preferred option in the older patient with overall lower demands on the hand. The main arthroplasty procedures for both osteoarthritis and rheumatoid arthritis are:

1. Suspension arthroplasty of 1st CMC joint (excision of trapezium).
2. Implant arthroplasty of the 1st CMC joint.
3. Implant arthroplasty of PIP joint.
4. Implant arthroplasty of MCP joint(s).

Suspension arthroplasty of 1st CMC joint (excision of trapezium)

Excisional arthroplasty has a long history and gives good pain relief and a mobile thumb (Froimson, 1970). Many surgeons now prefer this soft tissue procedure as it eliminates the risk

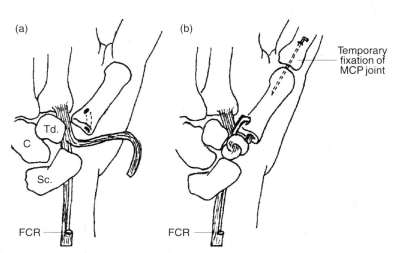

Figure 14.6. (a) Suspension arthroplasty involves excision of the trapezium and ligamentous reconstruction using a slip of the FCR tendon. (b) The slip of tendon is used both to reinforce the ligamentous suspension and to fill the cavity left by the removal of the trapezium. The MCP joint is sometimes held in slight flexion with a K-wire for a short period after surgery. Where hyperextension of the MCP joint is a problem, permanent stabilization by capsulodesis or fusion is indicated.

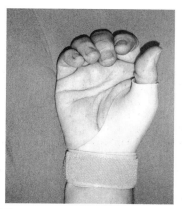

Figure 14.7. The thumb and wrist are immobilized for 6 weeks. The wrist is held in neutral or slight extension and the thumb is held in about 50 degrees of palmar abduction and 30 degrees of MCP joint flexion. The thumb IP joint is left free and should be exercised regularly throughout the day.

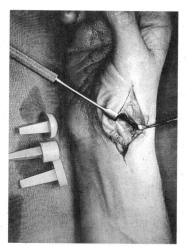

Figure 14.8. The trapezium is replaced by either a silicone elastomer implant (Swanson) or one of the newer implants which eliminate the problem of silicone particulate synovitis.

associated with silicone synovitis. The procedure involves excision of the trapezium and ligamentous reconstruction to prevent metacarpal displacement (Fig. 14.6).

A slip of the FCR tendon is used both to reinforce the ligamentous suspension and to fill the cavity left by the removal of the trapezium. The MCP joint may need to be stabilized by capsulodesis or arthrodesis as indicated.

A complication of this procedure is migration of the metacarpal. If there is proximal migration, a painful pseudoarthrosis can develop between the metacarpal and the distal end of the scaphoid. Radial displacement of the metacarpal can result in an adducted thumb.

Aftercare

Following surgery, the thumb and wrist are immobilized for 6 weeks with the wrist held in neutral or slight extension and the thumb in about 50 degrees of palmar abduction and 30 degrees of MCP joint flexion. Full movement of the thumb IP joint is allowed. On removal of the splint, gentle active CMC joint movements and light unresisted activity can be commenced. Normal use of the hand can usually be resumed 12 weeks after surgery (Fig. 14.7).

Implant arthroplasty of the 1st CMC joint

The trapezium is replaced by either a silicone elastomer implant (Swanson, 1972b) or one of the

newer implants which eliminate the problem of silicone particulate synovitis (Fig. 14.8). The main complication of implant arthroplasty is dislocation. This can be prevented by careful repair of the capsule and capsuloligamentous reinforcement using a strip of tendon, the most common being flexor carpi radialis. The MCP joint should be assessed for hyperextension deformity as this increases the tendency toward lateral and dorsal subluxation of the implant. A mild deformity can usually be corrected with a short period of K-wire fixation (2 to 3 weeks) following correction of the basal joint deformity. If the deformity is quite marked, i.e. greater than 25 degrees, it can be corrected with fusion or proximal advancement of the volar plate.

Aftercare

Postoperative management is the same as for suspension arthroplasty. Complications that can occur with this procedure include: radial neuritis or neuroma, radial artery damage, risk of infection with the introduction of a large foreign body or dislocation of the prosthesis.

Implant arthroplasty of the PIP joint

Adequate bone, soft tissue cover and an intact flexor/extensor mechanism are prerequisites for a successful outcome following this procedure. Patient selection is important. Young active patients requiring a strong grip and engaging in heavy

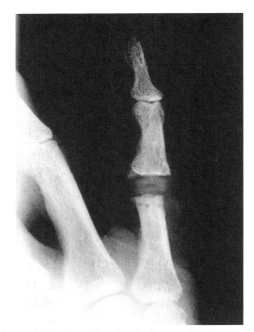

Figure 14.9. X-ray showing implant arthroplasty of the right little finger PIP joint in a 52-year-old man who had had post-traumatic arthritis for some years with gradual loss of joint flexibility. He was keen to restore flexion to the little finger so that he could continue his passion for playing golf.

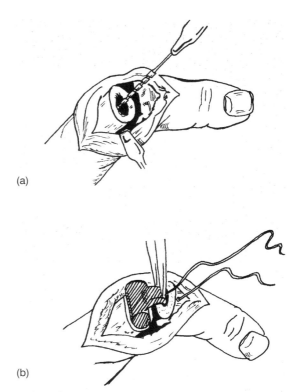

(a)

(b)

Figure 14.10. (a) The head of the proximal phalanx is resected and spurs are removed from the base of the middle phalanx. The medullary canals of both phalanges are reamed in a rectangular shape to take the implant. (b) The implant is inserted and the ligaments are reattached to the proximal phalanx with appropriate tension to provide good lateral stability and alignment.

manual labour are not suitable candidates for implant arthroplasty. Because of lateral stresses imposed on the index finger during pinch grip activity, PIP joint implant arthroplasty is less suitable for this digit. This procedure is generally indicated for the isolated disability of the middle, ring or little finger (Berger et al., 1999) (Fig. 14.9).

Implant arthroplasty of the PIP joint is occasionally indicated for the rheumatoid patient with severe swan-neck or boutonnière deformity. Reconstruction of the extensor mechanism will then be necessary.

Surgical technique

The joint is approached from either the dorsal or volar aspect depending on whether or not flexor tendon surgery is indicated. To expose the joint, the collateral ligaments and palmar plate are released proximally. The head of the proximal phalanx is resected and spurs are removed from the base of the middle phalanx. The medullary canals of both phalanges are reamed in a rectangular shape to take the implant. Following implant insertion, the

ligaments are reattached to the proximal phalanx with appropriate tension to provide good lateral stability and alignment (Fig. 14.10).

Aftercare

The aftercare regimen will depend on whether or not there has been tendon reconstruction to correct a swan-neck or boutonnière deformity. The most important postoperative considerations are:

1. Protective splinting of the joint for 6 weeks to avoid lateral deviation.
2. Early commencement of gentle active and passive flexion/extension exercises, i.e. 3 to 5 days after surgery in the absence of extensor tendon reconstruction (usually for RA).

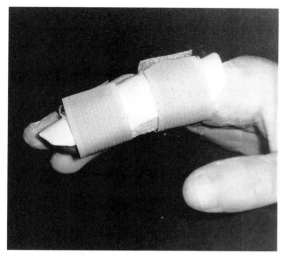

Figure 14.11. On the 2nd or 3rd postoperative day, the plaster cast is replaced with a dorsal thermoplastic finger splint that holds the digit in extension (except following swan-neck correction).

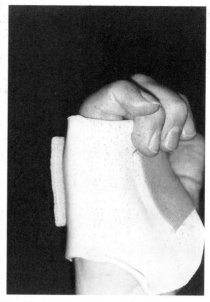

Figure 14.12. An MCP joint blocking splint can help concentrate flexion force at the PIP joint if the patient is overusing intrinsic muscles and 'hyperflexing' the MCP joints. It may also be necessary to block the DIP joint in extension with a small dorsal splint to maximize flexion at the PIP joint (not shown).

Where there has been extensor tendon reconstruction for swan-neck or boutonnière deformity, active movement is delayed for 10 days. Following correction of a swan-neck deformity, the PIP joint is maintained in 15 degrees of flexion throughout the 6-week splinting period. Following correction of a boutonnière deformity, the PIP joint is maintained in neutral extension.

The postoperative plaster cast is replaced by a dorsal thermoplastic finger splint 2 to 3 days after surgery. The splint should hold the PIP joint in neutral extension (other than for correction of swan-neck deformity) and reach midlaterally on both sides of the digit to prevent lateral movement. It should also include the DIP joint (Fig. 14.11).

Oedema control

Postoperative digital swelling is usually marked and can be addressed with a single layer of 2.5 cm Coban wrap used over the dressing. This is applied with great caution to avoid lateral stress to the PIP joint. Coban should only be applied by the therapist during the treatment session rather than by relatives at home. It is important that the splint is fitted following Coban application otherwise the splint will be too tight. A liberal coating of powder over the Coban will prevent the heated thermoplastic material from adhering to the wrap during moulding. The dorsal finger splint will usually

need to be remade after several days as swelling subsides.

Exercise protocol

In the absence of extensor tendon reconstruction, gentle active and passive flexion and extension exercises are commenced 3 to 5 days following surgery. These can be performed within the splint by simply releasing the distal strap. The patient should attempt 6 to 10 active and active-assisted repetitions every 2 to 3 hours during the 1st week of exercise. If the splint is removed for exercise, all fingers are flexed and extended together to provide lateral stability. By the 2nd week, exercise sessions can be performed 1 to 2 hourly with 10 to 15 repetitions.

To maximize PIP joint motion, it is sometimes necessary to immobilize the DIP joint in extension using a thin thermoplastic material to avoid bulkiness during active flexion exercises. An MCP joint blocking splint is effective if the patient is overusing intrinsic musculature; this will be evident if efforts to move the PIP joint result in hyperflexion of the MCP joints (Fig. 14.12).

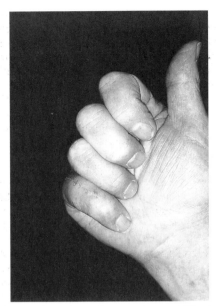

Figure 14.13. The 52-year-old patient (see Figure 14.9) obtained 70 degrees of active PIP joint flexion range within two weeks of surgery. He was fitted with a gentle dynamic hand-based flexion splint in the 3rd postoperative week when some tightening over the dorsum of the joint was becoming evident. The patient was advised to maintain passive and active flexion exercises and intermittent flexion splinting for at least a year after surgery.

Anticipated flexion range

Flexion range of the PIP joint following arthroplasty is in the vicinity of 70 degrees. With consistent effort, the patient can usually achieve this range within 2 weeks of surgery (Fig. 14.13). Where stiffness is a problem, a hand-based dynamic PIP flexion splint is used intermittently throughout the day. At all other times, the dorsal splint is used throughout the 6-week postoperative period.

Flexion range is readily lost if the patient does not persevere with the exercise/splinting regimen. Some patients have a greater propensity to stiffness; however, all patients are advised to maintain their home programme for at least a year.

Light activity is begun following splint removal. For protection during activity in weeks 6 to 12, the digit can be buddy-strapped to an adjacent finger to provide greater lateral stability.

Implant arthroplasty of MCP joint(s)

Implant arthroplasty of the MCP joints can be used for a single post-traumatic joint or to replace joints

which have been destroyed by rheumatoid disease (Fig. 14.14).

Surgical technique

Through a dorsal transverse incision, a soft tissue release of the joints is performed. The lateral ligaments and volar plate are usually released proximally and remain attached distally. The head of each metacarpal is resected. The metacarpal and phalangeal intramedullary canals are reamed to accept the appropriately sized implant. To avoid extensor tendon lag, the extensor tendon is reefed longitudinally.

Aim of postoperative management

The aim of postoperative treatment is to gain a balance between healing and the application of controlled motion so that the newly forming capsule will permit flexion/extension while simultaneously providing lateral and rotational stability. The deposition and remodelling of collagen around the implant will vary from patient to patient. The programme of prolonged splinting and early movement will therefore need to be tailored to the individual patient.

Immediate aftercare

The hand is maintained in its postoperative plaster for the first 2 to 3 days in elevation. This is achieved either with pillows or a non-constrictive sling. Careful attention is given to the alignment of the fingers to ensure that they do not rest in ulnar deviation. Small gauze squares are placed between

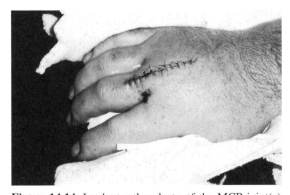

Figure 14.14. Implant arthroplasty of the MCP joint(s) can be used for a single post-traumatic joint (such as in the case of this 48-year-old man who sustained a crush injury) or to replace joints which have been destroyed by rheumatoid disease.

the digits to help maintain a slightly radial position. Cold packs can be used to help manage oedema and to alleviate pain. Gentle shoulder and elbow exercises are carried out regularly throughout the day.

On the 2nd postoperative day, active and active assisted MCP joint flexion and extension exercises are commenced. The fingers are moved in a pain-free range as a single unit to maintain correct alignment. The exercises are practised 5 to 10 times every 2 to 3 hours. When the patient has achieved a good range of intrinsic MCP joint flexion range, global flexion can be attempted, i.e., simultaneous flexion of the MCP, PIP and DIP joints.

Dynamic extension outrigger

On the 3rd or 4th postoperative day when oedema has subsided and some wound healing has occurred, the hand is fitted with a dorsal dynamic extension splint which is used during the day. The splint holds the wrist in 25 to 30 degrees of extension. Finger slings are placed on the proximal phalanges and hold the MCP joints in neutral extension with gentle elastic band traction (Fig. 14.15). The slings should place the digits in a slightly radial orientation to help prevent recurrence of ulnar drift. A resting splint is used for greater comfort at night.

Exercise protocol

Active MCP flexion exercises, with 5 to 10 repetitions, are performed hourly against the gentle tension of the rubber bands which will then return the joints to neutral extension. The tension of these

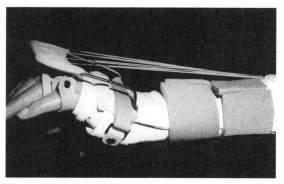

Figure 14.15. A dorsal dynamic extension outrigger is fitted 3 to 4 days postoperatively. Finger slings are worn on the proximal phalanges and hold the MCP joints in neutral extension with gentle elastic band traction.

bands is monitored daily for signs of fatigue and adjustments are made as necessary. Particular attention is given to the flexion range of the ring and little fingers. Full flexion of the index and middle fingers is less critical to grip function. The patient is encouraged to aim for 45 to 60 degrees of flexion at the index/middle fingers and 70 degrees of flexion at the ring/little fingers. If this cannot be achieved with relative ease, removing the slings of the ulnar two fingers during exercises may be necessary to gain a greater flexion range.

If attempts at active MCP joint flexion result in a 'hook' grip from overuse of the extrinsic flexors, it will be necessary to immobilize the interphalangeal joints in extension with small finger splints so that the flexion force can be transmitted through the MCP joints. When this difficulty has been overcome, global (or composite) flexion is attempted.

The reconstructed joint will begin to 'tighten' during the 2nd postoperative week. Movement not gained prior to this time will be difficult to achieve. It is therefore important that the patient is seen regularly during these early weeks so that progress can be monitored.

Sutures are removed at 2 weeks and gentle oil massage to the scar is commenced. A layer of Opsite Flexifix film or Hypafix will help flatten the scar as well as prevent irritation by the splint.

Dynamic MCP joint flexion splinting

A dynamic MCP joint flexion splint can be used intermittently throughout the day from the 3rd week onward to help overcome joint tightness. The extension outrigger and night splint are worn at all other times until the 6th postoperative week when the hand can be used for light daily activity. Some surgeons prefer to maintain the outrigger and night splint for a 12-week period. Lightly resisted activity is commenced at 8 weeks and gradually upgraded.

Intermittent dynamic flexion splinting may need to be maintained for some months following surgery. Decisions on just how long the splinting/exercise regimen should be maintained are made on a case by case basis (Fig. 14.16).

Rheumatoid arthritis

Rheumatoid disease is the most common of the connective tissue disorders. It is a systemic disease and is really an inflammatory synovitis rather than an arthritis (Ferlic et al., 1983).

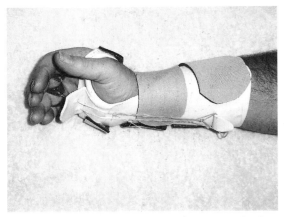

Figure 14.16. A dynamic MCP joint flexion splint is used intermittently after the 3rd postoperative week when tightness over the dorsum of the joint(s) usually becomes apparent.

The pathogenesis of RA is thought to be an immunological response occurring in the synovial tissues. The inflammatory synovium forms a pannus which grows over and infiltrates cartilage, tendons and ligaments and can result in:

1. Stretching of the joint capsule.
2. Erosion of cartilage and subchondral bone.
3. Disruption of ligamentous insertions.
4. Impaired tendon glide.
5. Nerve compression when present in closed compartments, e.g., the carpal tunnel.

These factors combine to cause pain, stiffness and deformity. Rheumatoid disease can also be associated with skin and pulmonary nodules, purpura, vasculitis and intrinsic muscle fibrosis.

Stages of rheumatoid disease

Rheumatoid arthritis can be divided into four clinical phases, the timing of which will vary from patient to patient:

1. Synovitis of joint and tendon mechanisms resulting in pain and swelling; no deformity is seen at this early stage. However, tendon glide may be impaired and crepitant.
2. Joint subluxation and/or dislocation is seen together with synovitis; the deformity can be passively corrected.
3. The deformity has become fixed; no joint destruction.
4. Joint destruction is evident.

Principles and types of management

Management of the rheumatoid patient requires a multidisciplinary approach involving several or all of the following health professionals: family physician, rheumatologist, surgeon, therapists, social worker and orthotist (Sones, 1971).

Because rheumatoid arthritis is not a static condition, evaluation and treatment are an ongoing process. Involvement of hand structures cannot be viewed in isolation because the disabling effects of this disease are manifold, usually involving numerous joints and other tissues or organs. The psychological and social implications of this chronic and disabling condition also need to be considered in the overall assessment.

Medical management

Drug therapy is the first line of defence used to control the disease process. Drugs used in treatment include salicylates, steroids, gold, antimalarials, cytotoxics (methotrexate) and immunosuppressants. Each may be effective for a particular patient; however, every drug can have significant side effects and patient response and dosage must be carefully monitored and regulated.

Therapy

Many patients now diagnosed with rheumatoid disease are well controlled with the newer drug regimens and may have little need of therapy intervention. In those patients not responding well to medication and where pain, stiffness and deformity are troublesome, the goals of therapy are:

1. To provide support to painful joints with night and intermittent day splinting.
2. To maintain and/or increase joint mobility with gentle active and active assisted movements performed in a pain-free range.
3. To maintain and/or improve muscle strength with isometric exercise.
4. To determine functional problems and recommend aids to daily living and modifications to the patient's home-work-leisure environment.
5. To teach the patient joint protection techniques and provide information about the disease.

Apart from providing support to painful, inflamed joints, splints are sometimes used to place the wrist, thumb or digits in a more functional position, e.g. a soft splint to correct ulnar drift of the fingers will sometimes enhance pinch grip function. It should be noted, however, that splints do not reverse deformities and probably do little to prevent further deterioration of an already existing deformity.

Deformities of the rheumatoid hand

Dorsal subluxation of the ulnar head

This is characterized by a prominent ulnar head. Wrist synovitis generally begins in the ulnar carpus, stretching the ulnar carpal ligaments and the triangular fibrocartilaginous complex (TFCC). The consequences of this are three-fold and are known as the 'caput ulna syndrome':

1. The distal ulna dislocates dorsally.
2. The carpus supinates in relation to the hand.
3. The ECU tendon subluxes volarly.

These factors result in painful and restricted forearm rotation, loss of wrist extension and a radially deviated wrist from the unopposed ECRL and ECRB muscles. Attrition ruptures of the ulnar extensor tendons are commonly associated with this syndrome which is seen in about a third of patients with rheumatoid disease.

Collapse deformity of the wrist

This deformity is characterized by radial deviation of the metacarpals and concomitant ulnar deviation

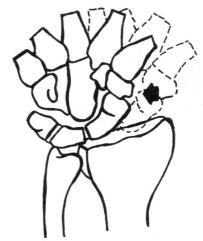

Figure 14.18. Ulnar translocation of the carpus involves the radiocarpal ligaments which have undergone the attritional effects of chronic synovitis. The carpus translocates ulnarly due to ligament insufficiency. (Reproduced from Garcia-Elias, M. Carpal instabilities and dislocations. In *Green's Operative Hand Surgery* (D. P. Green, R. N. Hotchkiss and W. C. Pederson, eds) p. 873, Churchill Livingstone, with permission.)

of the MCP joints. It involves the radiocarpal ligaments, the destruction of which results in scapholunate dissociation and rotational instability of the scaphoid (volarly) and the lunate (dorsally). The subsequent loss of carpal height results in an imbalance in the extensor tendon mechanism. This collapse deformity is thought to be responsible for the recurrence of ulnar drift of the fingers following MCP joint arthroplasty (Fig. 14.17).

Ulnar translocation of the carpus

This deformity also involves the radiocarpal ligaments which have undergone the attritional effects of chronic synovitis. This resultant ligament insufficiency can cause the carpus to slide down the radius and translocate ulnarly (Fig. 14.18).

Volar subluxation/dislocation of the MCP joints and ulnar drift of the fingers

The finger MCP joints are particularly vulnerable to the deforming forces of rheumatoid disease because they allow motion in two planes and are therefore less stable (Fig. 14.19).

The aetiology of MCP joint deformity involves wrist pathology, tendon forces, imbalance of

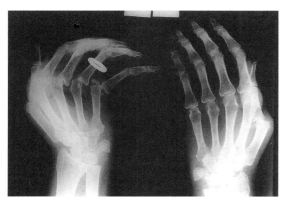

Figure 14.17. Collapse deformity of the wrist is characterized by radial deviation of the metacarpals and concomitant ulnar deviation at the MCP joints. Note the erosion at the MCP joints.

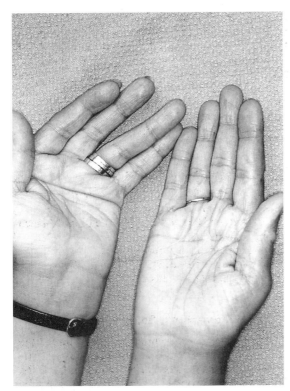

Figure 14.19. Ulnar drift of the fingers is a common deformity in rheumatoid disease.

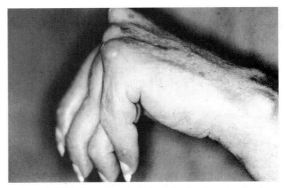

Figure 14.20. Swan-neck deformity is characterized by PIP joint hyperextension and DIP joint flexion. With the MCP joints locked into a flexed position, the intrinsic muscles exert a greater force through the central extensor tendon. Because the PIP joint capsule and volar plate are already stretched from the disease process, hyperextension of the PIP joints readily ensues.

intrinsic musculature and the effects of gravity and pinch grip force. The extensor mechanism is stretched as a result of chronic synovitis causing the tendons to slip ulnarly. Flexor tendon forces can further stretch already compromised volar capsular and ligamentous structures.

Boutonnière (button-hole) deformity

This deformity is characterized by flexion of the PIP joint and hyperextension of the DIP and MCP joints. Due to proliferative synovitis, the central extensor tendon is weakened, lengthened and may rupture. The extension force of the tendon is therefore diminished. The lateral bands fall below the axis of the joint, flexing rather than extending it. There is secondary shortening of the oblique retinacular ligament which results in DIP joint hyperextension and limited active flexion of this joint. Hyperextension of the MCP joints results from compensatory efforts to extend the PIP joint. In the early stages, this deformity is passively

correctable. As the joint capsule gradually contracts, the deformity becomes fixed.

Swan-neck deformity

This deformity is characterized by PIP joint hyperextension and DIP joint flexion. The deformity can originate at either the PIP or DIP joint (Fig. 14.20). Where there is flexor tendon synovitis, difficulty in initiating finger flexion with the extrinsic flexors may result in excessive flexion effort being transmitted through the MCP joints via the intrinsic musculature. With the MCP joints in this flexed position, the intrinsic muscles are able to exert a greater force through the central extensor tendon and if the PIP joint volar capsule and palmar plate are stretched as a result of the disease process, hyperextension at this joint readily ensues. As the deformity develops, the lateral bands slip dorsally, further accentuating hyperextension of the PIP joint with reciprocal flexion at the DIP joint.

Where there is elongation or rupture of the distal extensor tendon, the swan-neck deformity can be secondary to a mallet-type deformity.

Thumb

Like the fingers, the thumb can develop a boutonnière or swan-neck deformity. In the case of the former, the primary problem lies with synovitis of the MCP joint. In the case of the latter, the primary

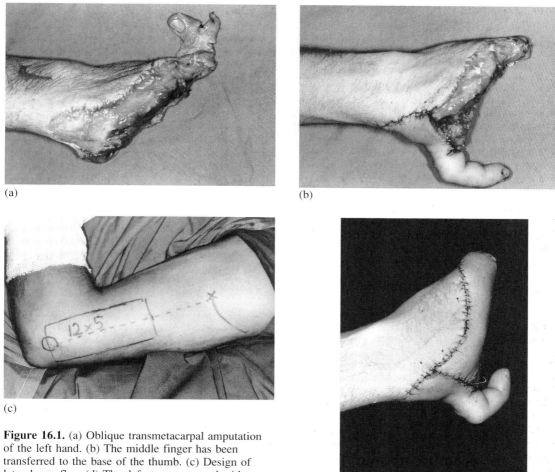

Figure 16.1. (a) Oblique transmetacarpal amputation of the left hand. (b) The middle finger has been transferred to the base of the thumb. (c) Design of lateral arm flap. (d) The defect was covered with a fasciocutaneous lateral arm flap.

consists of the lateral aspect of the great toe and the medial aspect of the second toe. It is supplied by the first dorsal metatarsal artery (FDMA), a branch of the dorsalis pedis artery, or the first plantar metatarsal artery. Its innervation is through both the deep peroneal nerve and the medial plantar nerve. The main advantage of the first web space flap for sensory reconstruction in the hand is replacement of pulp skin with similar thin, glabrous skin with concentrated sensory receptors. This allows the best chance for restoration of functional sensibility.

The toes are the source of many free flaps for reconstruction of the hand. Thumb loss, especially at, or proximal to, the MCP joint, can be reconstructed with a free, whole great toe, or second

toe. The second and third toes can be used to reconstruct missing fingers in certain congenital and post-traumatic conditions (Fig. 16.2). Vascularized toe joint transfers have been used to replace destroyed PIP and MCP joints; however, the longevity of these reconstructions remains to be seen.

Fascial flaps

Because some of the commonly used fasciocutaneous flaps are either too fat for dorsal hand reconstruction or leave an unacceptable donor site scar, the search for a tissue source that avoids these problems was undertaken. Fascial flaps satisfy both these requirements. They have several advantages:

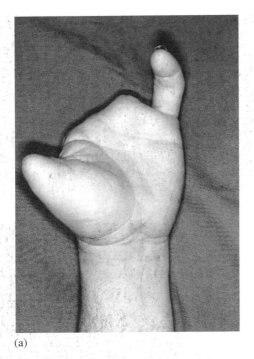

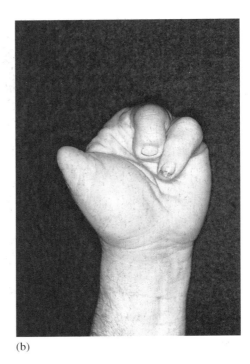

(a)   (b)

Figure 16.2. (a) Defect resulting from a fan blade injury to the left hand. (b) A good functional result was achieved following transfer of the second toe to the ring finger.

1. They provide thin, pliable cover without bulk.
2. They are readily contoured to the defect.
3. For the most part, they leave an inconspicuous donor site scar.
4. They are useful where a gliding surface is required for tendons and nerves.

Fascial flaps are used most commonly for defects on the dorsum of the hand, the volar hand and wrist and in the first web space, especially following release of extensive contractures.

The only problems with these flaps is their relatively limited size and the fact that they require a skin graft to cover them. Occasionally, skin graft 'take' can be variable due to haematoma formation beneath them.

The temporoparietal fascia can be harvested as a free flap, taking a piece of tissue as large as 14×10 cm. The donor site is hidden beneath the hair and providing that care is taken during elevation of the flap, alopecia should not be a problem. The radial and ulnar forearm flaps and the lateral arm flap can also be raised as fascial flaps only, leaving a linear donor site scar.

Aftercare following fascial flaps

Following free fascial flaps, the area is rested for the 1st postoperative week after which gentle movement is begun. To prevent hypertrophic scarring, pressure therapy, e.g. silicone scar gel, is instituted after 3 weeks.

Muscle flaps

The malleability of muscle flaps makes them well suited to difficult contour problems in the upper extremity. This is especially the case in large, post-traumatic defects (Fig. 16.3).

Muscle flaps have a better vascularity than fasciocutaneous flaps and are more readily able to deliver antibiotics to infected, or potentially infected wounds. For this reason, they are useful in the management of chronic osteomyelitis.

The muscle selected will be determined by the size and contour of the defect. For small defects, the serratus anterior is useful as it has a long pedicle and minimal donor site morbidity. Similarly, gracilis is useful in long, thin defects.

The hand may also be discoloured, i.e. red, blue or purple, and often has a mottled appearance. This becomes more marked when the hand is dependent and often reverses dramatically when the hand is then elevated. Distinct red areas are sometimes present over the dorsum of the index and middle finger MCP joints.

5. Trophic changes

These changes involve skin, nails, hair and bone. The skin frequently has a glossy appearance resulting from nutritional changes. The fat pads at the tips of the fingers atrophy, causing the nails to curve downward, thus giving a 'pencil-pointing' appearance. Flattening of the cuticle base and rugae pattern may be observed. The nails can become thickened and rigid and the hair may coarsen.

Osteoporosis results from demineralization and becomes evident on X-rays at about the 5th week. In the early stages of the disease, osteoporosis is seen in the polar region of the long bones, i.e. the metacarpal and phalangeal bones. In advanced cases of CRPS, osteoporosis is evident in the carpal bones.

Possible triggers of CRPS

While CRPS can result from a trivial injury, there are certain injuries, surgical procedures or irritation of specific nerves that result in a higher incidence of this condition. They include:

1. Distal radial fractures which frequently affect the median nerve and require prolonged cast immobilization.
2. Carpal tunnel decompression where there can be injury to the palmar cutaneous branch of the median nerve.
3. Decompression of the first dorsal compartment for de Quervain's syndrome where there can be injury to the superficial branch of the radial nerve.
4. Palmar fasciectomy for Dupuytren's disease (incidence of about 7 per cent in Australia).
5. Injury to the dorsal branch of the ulnar nerve during procedures involving the distal ulna or from trauma to this area.
6. Digital amputations with neuroma formation.

Patient presentation

Whilst this condition can occur in patients ranging in age from the late teens to the elderly, the average age is 45 years. Women develop this condition three times more often than men. There is a statistical relationship to smoking. This syndrome can be confined to a single digit, involve the whole hand and occasionally, the entire upper limb.

It can sometimes be difficult to distinguish the signs and symptoms of a CRPS from those that accompany any significant hand trauma.

The therapist should suspect the onset of CRPS if:

1. Symptoms of pain, stiffness and swelling do not begin to subside after several weeks of hand therapy.
2. There is a sudden increase in the above symptoms that cannot readily be explained, e.g. by overuse of the hand on the previous day. Hand oedema that worsens in the early evening and subsides by morning can also be an indicator.
3. The patient suddenly exhibits or reports signs or symptoms that have been previously absent, e.g. sensations of burning or heat, mottling of the skin, excessive sweating or swelling that cannot be accounted for.
4. A patient who has not had nerve damage reports altered sensory perception, e.g. when touching the face or hair, the patient will describe the texture as being 'rough' in comparison to the unaffected hand.

Diagnostic testing

The diagnosis of CRPS is usually made on clinical findings. Investigations that can help confirm the diagnosis include:

1. X-ray which will show osteoporosis after the 5th week (Bickerstaff et al., 1991).
2. Bone scan.
3. The 'skin wrinkle test' for the assessment of sympathetic function (Vasudevan et al., 2000).
4. Diagnostic blocks such as a stellate ganglion or somatic nerve block. A positive response will indicate that pain is being sympathetically maintained and that the use of oral sympatholytic drugs is indicated.

Treatment

The patient with CRPS is generally managed best by a team approach. The members of this team should include: the specialist, the patient's family practitioner, a pain specialist (anaesthetist) and a hand therapist. Most cases of CRPS will reverse quite quickly after suitable treatment strategies have been instituted. Where the condition is prolonged and is impacting on the patient's coping mechanisms and affecting family/work dynamics, the inclusion of a psychologist and rehabilitation consultant may be warranted. There are commonly three components to patient management:

1. Hand therapy.
2. Pharmacological intervention (non-invasive and invasive).
3. Psychological support.

In a small number of patients, surgery may be indicated.

Hand therapy

The hand therapist has frequent and close contact with the patient and is often the first to recognise the signs and symptoms of CRPS. If the specialist favours a conservative approach to management, the patient will be started on transcutaneous nerve stimulation (TENS) and the active 'stress-loading programme' described by Watson and Carlson (1987). If the response to TENS is favourable, the patient is loaned a unit for home use. The therapy protocol will need to address the entire upper limb to avoid restriction of shoulder movement from secondary adhesive capsulitis.

The 'stress-loading' programme comprises traction and compression exercises that provide stressful stimuli to the extremity without joint motion. This programme has been used for 30 years. It is simple to execute, non-invasive and appropriately places some onus of care onto the patient.

Until pain, swelling and autonomic signs have abated, all other hand therapy treatment modalities are delayed. Prior to commencement of the programme, the patient is warned that increased pain and swelling are a typical response for the first few days and generally settle.

Method

The 'compression' exercise requires a scrubbing brush. The patient assumes the quadruped position. The scrubbing brush is held in the affected hand and the patient begins scrubbing a smooth surface such as plywood board using a backward-forward motion. The patient should lean over the arm and maintain elbow extension (Fig. 18.3).

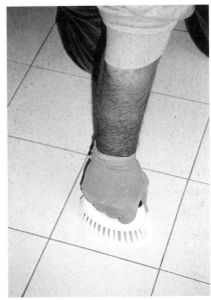

Figure 18.3. The 'compression' component of the 'stress-loading' programme involves the patient assuming the quadruped position and scrubbing a smooth surface using a backward-forward motion with the elbow extended and the patient leaning over the arm. This motion is initially performed for 3 minutes, three times a day.

Where it is impractical or difficult for the patient to assume this position, scrubbing can be performed on a tabletop. The motion should be continued for 3 minutes and be performed three times daily. After several days, the sessions are increased to 5 minutes, and then to 7 minutes after a fortnight. The upgrading of the programme should be commensurate with the patient's ability to cope.

The 'traction' component of the programme is achieved by carrying a lightly weighted bag whenever the patient is standing or walking. For ease of grasp, rubber insulation tubing can be cut and taped over the handles of a disposable plastic bag. The tubing provides an enlarged, comfortable and slip-resistant 'handle'. The initial weight in the bag is approximately 0.5 kg; this is gradually increased to a 2.5 kg weight (Fig. 18.4).

Other therapy measures

When pain has begun to subside, appropriate therapy measures to overcome residual oedema and stiffness are commenced. These measures are

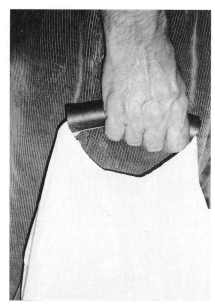

Figure 18.4. The 'traction' component of the programme involves carrying a lightly weighted bag whenever standing or walking. For ease of grasp, insulation tubing is cut open and taped over the handles of a disposable plastic bag.

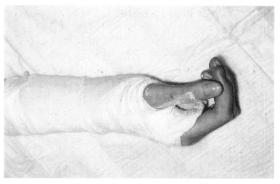

Figure 18.5. Where wrist stiffness is a problem, serial plaster splinting to restore extension is important to facilitate finger flexion.

introduced gradually and response to them is assessed to avoid exacerbation of the condition.

Pressure garments

Pressure gloves or compression wraps for oedema are used cautiously as they frequently aggravate pain and/or swelling. They should be worn for short periods initially, i.e. 15 to 30 minutes. If there is no adverse response, the wearing time is increased.

Exercise

Exercise should commence with active rather than passive motion as the latter often provokes pain. When passive exercise is commenced, it is best performed by the patient rather than the therapist.

If wrist stiffness is a problem, priority is given to regaining extension so that finger flexion can be optimized. The wrist can be serially splinted using a volar plaster which is held in place with a crepe bandage. A wrist that is comfortably supported is also less painful (Fig. 18.5).

The exercise regimen should be performed hourly and include all upper limb joints. Repeated active movement of the more proximal joints cannot be overemphasized. Exercise involving the fingers and thumb should be carried out in a sustained and systematic fashion with emphasis on stabilized interphalangeal joint exercises.

Splinting

The MCP joints are frequently stiff and may require a dynamic flexion splint. Interphalangeal joint finger stiffness can be overcome by gently bandaging the hand into flexion with a wide crepe bandage and immersing the hand in warm water for 15-minute periods several times a day. This combination of stretch and warmth is highly effective in increasing joint flexibility prior to active finger flexion exercises.

Opsite Flexifix

Over the past 18 months, the author has been using Opsite Flexifix to help manage the causalgic pain that many CRPS patients experience (Boscheinen-Morrin and Shannon, 2000). The use of Opsite in this way follows from a study carried out by the King's College Hospital in London (Foster et al., 1994). It concluded that Opsite used on unbroken skin in diabetics was effective in relieving the pain of peripheral neuropathy. The Opsite is applied to those areas of the hand which are most symptomatic (Fig. 18.6).

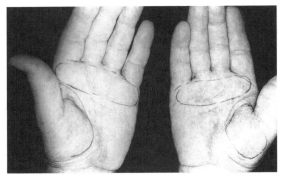

Figure 18.6. To help relieve the 'burning' sensations in this gentleman's hands following bilateral open carpal tunnel decompression, Opsite Flexifix was applied to the reddened areas of discomfort. The area of application is outlined.

Functional activity

The patient is encouraged to use the affected hand in appropriate normal daily activity. Activity is carefully upgraded in accordance with the patient's progress. The 'stress-loading' programme can be scaled back as improvement is noted. The time-frame of management will vary from patient to patient; however, the programme should be reinstituted at the first sign that symptoms of CRPS may be recurring.

Psychological implications

Chronic regional pain syndrome is a distressing condition. Apart from the physical discomfort, the patient is unable to engage in normal work and recreational activities and relationships with family and friends soon become strained. These patients frequently become depressed if the condition persists for more than a few weeks. If this is the case, referral to a psychologist or psychiatrist is indicated.

Pharmacological treatment

The pharmacological approach to managing CRPS is complex and under constant review (Czop et al., 1996). Drugs are often used in combination with one another or with intravenous regional sympathetic blocks.

The following categories of drugs are used:

1. Antidepressants – the most commonly used are the tricyclic group, e.g. Tofranil, Sinequan.
2. Anticonvulsants – e.g. Dilantin, Tegretol.
3. Membrane-stabilizing agents – e.g. Lidocaine.
4. Calcium channel blockers – such as Procardia and Norvasc which are arterial vasodilators.
5. Corticosteroids – e.g. prednisone.
6. Adrenergic compounds – such as Catapress and Dibenzyline.

As with any drug, patients need to be carefully screened for suitability prior to prescription and then monitored for potential side effects.

Regional intravenous sympathetic block

The Hannington-Kiff blockade (1974) for sympathetic pain is a modification of the analgesic drug infusion described by Bier in 1908. These blocks, using intravenous drugs such as guanethidine (Field et al., 1993), reserpine and bretylium tosylate, usually need to be repeated 3 to 5 times at 2 to 3 week intervals. Their therapeutic effect usually becomes apparent 2 to 3 days following infusion when hand therapy techniques can be employed with maximum efficacy. Guanethidine and reserpine are no longer available in the United States.

Surgery

When the clinical signs and symptoms of CRPS have settled, surgery may be necessary to correct the neural or mechanical trigger of the pain syndrome, i.e. a neuroma may require resection or the median nerve may require further decompression. Other patients may need to undergo release of secondary joint contractures. All surgical patients will require sympatholytic medication during and after surgery to avoid potential recurrence of their symptoms.

For patients with an entrenched pain syndrome, the place of chemical or surgical sympathectomy is controversial.

References

Bickerstaff, D. R., O'Doherty, D. P. and Kanis, J. A. (1991). Radiographic changes in algodystrophy of the hand. *J. Hand Surg.,* **16B**, 47–52.

Boscheinen-Morrin, J. and Shannon, J. (2000). Opsite Flexifix: an effective adjunct in the management of pain and hypersensitivity in the hand. *Aust. J. Occ. Ther.,* (submitted for publication).

Covington, E. C. (1995). Psychological issues in reflex sympathetic dystrophy. In *Reflex Sympathetic Dystrophy: A*

Reappraisal. Progress in Pain Research and Management. Vol. 6 (W. Jaenig and M. Stanton-Hicks, eds) pp. 191–215, IASP Press.

Czop, C., Smith, T. L., Rauck, R. and Koman, L. A. (1996). The pharmacologic approach to the painful hand. *Hand Clin., 12,* 633–42.

Field, J., Monk, C. and Atkins, R. M. (1993). Objective improvements in algodystrophy following regional intravenous guanethidine. *J. Hand Surg.,* **18B,** 339–42.

Foster, A. V. M., Eaton, C., McConville, D. O. and Edmonds, M. E. (1994). Application of Opsite film: a new and effective treatment of painful diabetic neuropthy. *Diab. Med.,* **11,** 768–72.

Jaenig, W. (1995). The puzzle of 'reflex sympathetic dystrophy': mechanisms, hypotheses, open questions. In *Reflex Sympathetic Dystrophy: A Reappraisal. Progress in Pain Research and Management.* Vol. 6 (W. Jaenig and M. Stanton-Hicks, eds) pp. 1–24, IASP Press.

Koman, L. A., Smith, T. L., Smith, B. P. and Li, Z. (1996). The painful hand. *Hand Clin.,* **12,** 757–64.

Koman, L. A., Poehling, G. G. and Smith, T. L. (1999). Complex regional pain syndrome: reflex sympathetic dystrophy and causalgia. In *Green's Operative Hand Surgery* (D. P. Green, R. N. Hotchkiss and W. C. Pederson, eds) pp. 636–66, Churchill Livingstone.

Merskey, H. and Bogduk, N. (1994). Classification of chronic pain. Descriptions of chronic pain syndromes and definitions of pain terms. *Prog. Pain Res. Management, 1,* 39–43.

Pollock, F. E. Jr., Koman, L. A., Smith, B. P. and Poehling, G. G. (1993). Patterns of microvascular response associated with reflex sympathetic dystrophy of the hand and wrist. *J. Hand Surg.,* **18A,** 847–52.

Watson, H. K. and Carlson, L. (1987). Treatment of reflex sympathetic dystrophy of the hand with an active 'stress loading' program. *J. Hand Surg.,* **12A,** 779–85.

Vasudevan, T. M., van Ru, A. M., Nukada, H. and Taylor, P. K. (2000). Skin wrinkling for the assessment of sympathetic function in the limbs. *Aust. N. Z. J. Surg.,* **70,** 57–9.

Further reading

Amadio, P. C., Mackinnon, S. E., Merritt, W. H., et al. (1991). Reflex sympathetic dystrophy syndrome: consensus report of an ad hoc committee of the American Association for Hand Surgery on the definition of reflex sympathetic dystrophy. *Plast. Reconstr. Surg.,* **87,** 371–5.

Atkins, R. M., Duckworth, T. and Kanis, J. A. (1990). Features of algodystrophy after Colles' fracture. *J. Bone Joint Surg.,* **72B,** 105–10.

Blanchard, J., Ramamurthy, S. Walsh, N., et al. (1990). Intravenous regional sympatholysis: a double-blind comparison of guanethidine, reserpine and normal saline. *J. Pain Symp. Management,* **5,** 357–61.

Boas, R. A. (1995). Complex regional pain syndromes: symptoms, signs and differential diagnosis. In *Reflex Sympathetic Dystrophy: A Reappraisal. Progress in Pain Research and Management* Vol. 6, (W.Janig and M. Stanton-Hicks, eds) pp. 79–92, IASP Press.

Bohm, E. (1978). Transcutaneous electrical nerve stimulation in chronic pain after peripheral nerve injury. *Acta Neurochir.,* **40,** 277–87.

Campbell, J. N., Raja, S. N., Selig, D. K., et al. (1994). Diagnosis and management of sympathetically maintained pain. *Prog. Pain Res. Management, 1,* 85–100.

Dobyns, J. H. (1991). Pain dysfunction syndrome. In *Operative Nerve Repair and Reconstruction* (R. H. Gelberman, ed.) pp. 1489–96, J. B. Lippincott.

Duncan, K. H., Lewis, R. C., Racz, G. and Nordyke, M. D. (1988). Treatment of upper extremity reflex sympathetic dystrophy with joint stiffness using sympatholytic Bier blocks and manipulation. *Orthopaedics, 11,* 883–6.

Feinmann, C. (1985). Pain relief by anti-depressants: possible modes of action. *Pain, 23,* 1–8.

Grundberg, A. B. (1996). Reflex sympathetic dystrophy: treatment with long-acting intramuscular corticosteroids. *J. Hand Surg.,* **21A,** 667–70.

Jupiter, J. B., Seiler, J. G. and Zienowicz, R. (1994). Sympathetic maintained pain (causalgia) associated with a demonstrable peripheral nerve lesion. *J. Bone Joint Surg.,* **76A,** 1376–84.

Melzack, R. (1975). Prolonged relief of pain by brief, intense, transcutaneous somatic stimulation. *Pain, 1,* 357–73.

Mullins, P. (1992). Reflex sympathetic dystrophy. In *Concepts in Hand Rehabilitation* (B. Stanley and S. Tribuzi, eds) F. A. Davis.

Ochoa, J. L. (1992). Reflex sympathetic dystrophy: a disease of medical understanding. *Clin. J. Pain,* **8,** 363–6.

Saplys, R., Mackinnon, S. E. and Dellon, A. L. (1987). The relationship between nerve entrapment versus neuroma complications and the misdiagnosis of de Quervain's disease. *Contemp. Orthop.,* **15,** 51–7.

Walsh, M. T. (1995). Therapist's management of reflex sympathetic dystrophy. In *Rehabilitation of the Hand: Surgery and Therapy* (J. M. Hunter, E. J. Mackin and A. D. Callahan, eds) pp. 817–33, Mosby.

Index